What others are saying about this book:

"As Chairman of the National Commission on Sleep Disorders, I have heard testimony from both men and women describing the disintegration of families, the financial ruin of successful individuals and death, caused by lack of refreshing sleep because of sleep apnea syndrome. It is imperative that the public be made more aware of this serious sleep problem."

> — *William C. Dement, M.D., Ph.D.*
> *Director, Sleep Disorder Clinic*
> *Stanford University School of Medicine*

"*Snoring Can Kill!!* should be must reading for everyone. It explains so clearly and quickly the frightening facts about this extremely serious sleep problem."

> — *Diana Guth, B.A., R.R.T., Chief Executive Officer,*
> *Home Respiratory Care Company*
> *Westwood, California*

"My dental practice involves the diagnosis and treatment of sleep disorders, and it is rare when I have the opportunity to recommend a book that has value as a guide to understanding a condition that plagues humanity. This book will be required reading for my patients."

> — *James F. Garry, D.D.S., F.I.C.D., F.I.C.C.M.O., F.A.A.H.D.*

"I have always been concerned about my husband's snoring, but just dismissed it as a normal occurrence. Thanks to *Snoring Can Kill!!* I understand so much more about the causes of his annoying nightly noises."

> — *Marsha Simonds*

"This book is a must for anyone concerned about snoring and fatigue! As a doctor with a serious snoring and sleep apnea problem, I urge you to read this concise, easy to understand book. My snoring is gone and I have much more energy and pep."

> — *Richard D. Price, M.D.*

Snoring Can Kill!!

Discover How Sleep Apnea Can Be Ruining Your Life

Joseph L. Goldstein

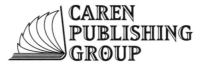

CAREN
PUBLISHING
GROUP

Pacific Palisades, California

The information and procedures contained in this book are based upon the research and personal experiences of the author. They are not intended as a substitute for consulting with your physician or other health care provider. The publisher and author are not responsible for any adverse effects or consequences resulting from the use of any suggestions or procedures discussed in this book or the resources listed in the appendixes. All matters pertaining to your physical health should be supervised by a health care professional.

©1999 Joseph Goldstein

Publisher's Cataloging-in-Publication
(Provided by Quality Books, Inc.)
Goldstein, Joseph L.
       Snoring can kill!! : discover how sleep apnea can
   be ruining your life!! / by Joseph L. Goldstein. —
   1st ed.
       p. cm.
       LCCN: 98-94827
       ISBN 0-9668939-5-6

       1. Sleep apnea syndromes—Popular works.
   2. Snoring. I. Title.

RC737.5/g65 1999   616.2
                                              QBI98-1722

Copyeditor: Barbara Coster, Cross-t.i Copyediting, Santa Barbara, California
Cover design: Karl Nayeri, Prime Graphics, Los Angeles, California
Interior illustrations: Louis LaRose, LaRose Graphics, Northridge, California
Book design: Christine Nolt, Cirrus Design, Santa Barbara, California

Printed in the United States of America.

To my beloved family,

Jill, Caren, Steven and Lois,

for enduring my nightly snoring

CONTENTS

Consider and answer me, O Lord, my God; lighten my eyes, lest I sleep the sleep of death.

— Psalm 13

Chapter 1

Please Note!

I am not a doctor, I am not even a health professional. I am a regular, everyday working person just like you who snores so loudly that my wife and I have been sleeping in separate bedrooms for over 20 years.

Believe me, just like every other problem snorer, I have been the butt of many snoring jokes and insults and always thought my snoring was harmless and perfectly normal.

Then one day I discovered that snoring was absolutely no joke and that I had a very serious medical problem that could eventually cause catastrophic problems to my well-being and quality of life.

This intentionally concise, easy to read, nontechnical, nonmedical book is intended to inform you of the very serious health risks and potentially deadly consequences of undiagnosed, untreated snoring. It explains how you can determine if you or someone in your family might require further medical diagnosis, what tests are available, and what to expect if you discover that you are a victim of this debilitating, life-threatening medical problem associated with your snoring.

Please note that I am not a doctor, and although my personal opinions will undoubtedly sneak in every once in a while, it is not my intention to give medical advice since I am not qualified to do so!

There are hundreds of excellent, more technical, medically oriented books available at any bookstore or library that go into greater detail on snoring and related sleep disorder problems with in-depth, complicated, scientific descriptions and terms. But my primary goal is to quickly present to the reader, in the most simple, easy to understand language, the basic facts about the potential dangers of snoring and to convince anyone who might feel they have the symptoms related to this problem to seek competent medical assistance immediately.

For the past several years, I have studied sleep disorders to learn more about my own snoring problems and have traveled worldwide to meet with the leading medical and dental experts in this field. The most important warning I can give is to be very careful of so-called cures for snoring.

In newspapers, on the radio and on TV, there are advertisements for miraculous laser and surgical medical procedures that might work well for normal snoring difficulties. But these same procedures could cause irreparable damage if the sufferer has more severe sleep disorder problems.

In addition, there are also many drugstore products and over-the-counter medications readily available without prescription that claim to eliminate or minimize snoring as well as other sleep disorders. But without proper medical advice and examination, these products and procedures may not be adequate or safe to relieve your particular snoring condition and could jeopardize your health.

If you feel that you might have a sleep-related problem that is affecting your quality of life and your happiness, I urge you to see a sleep specialist. It is absolutely essential to get competent medical advice from sleep disorder experts and to follow their recommendations faithfully to overcome the many day-to-day health problems and deadly medical risks that snoring-related sleep disorders can cause.

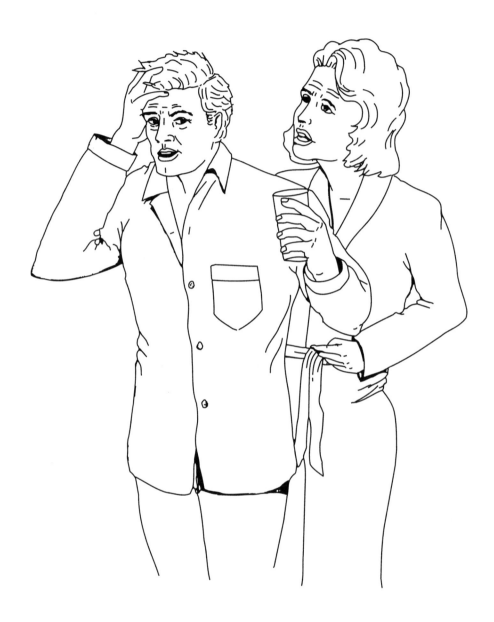

I would wake up every morning feeling miserable, tired
and sluggish without knowing the cause.

When I lie down, I say, When shall I arise, and the night be gone? And I am full of tossings to and fro unto the dawning of the day.

— Job 7.4

Chapter 2
Ruined Lives

Tomorrow morning, more than 30 million Americans will wake up feeling terrible. They will start the day tired and sluggish with a bad headache. They will be irritable and have a difficult time getting off to a good start. When they get to work, they will be drowsy and might even nap at their desk. As they drive home, they will have a difficult time staying awake or may actually fall asleep behind the wheel and be involved in a dangerous, life-threatening accident. At home, they will probably have an argument with the family and be cranky. All through the day they will try to pep themselves up with coffee or other stimulants to fight this distressing fatigue.

These same unfortunate sufferers will have sexual and marital problems, toss and turn during a restless night's sleep and get up many times during the night to go to the bathroom.

When and if they consult their doctor, there is a good possibility they will be misdiagnosed and told that their fatigue is caused by worry, a hormonal deficiency, lack of vitamins, or is just a normal part of growing old.

But the sad truth is that in many cases these symptoms are caused by a very harmful, life-threatening sleep disorder closely related to snoring called sleep apnea. If left undiagnosed and untreated, sleep apnea can be a deadly killer causing heart problems, stroke, high blood pressure, mental deterioration and a multitude of other unexplained physical problems.

I know full well about this problem and the miserable effects it can have on one's life. Because until November 22, 1996, I was an unknowing victim of sleep apnea and suffered the many dire consequences of this disorder without being aware of the reason for my feeling so depressed, tired and miserable even after what I considered to be a good night's sleep.

I would wake up in the morning feeling more tired than when I went to bed. I would have a pounding headache all morning until I took aspirin after aspirin to relieve the pain. I would lack energy and have a tough time getting along with people, especially my family. My job and family life were in trouble. I felt awful, miserable, depressed and constantly sleepy. For over 20 years I went from doctor to doctor describing how I felt and was repeatedly told by some of the finest doctors in

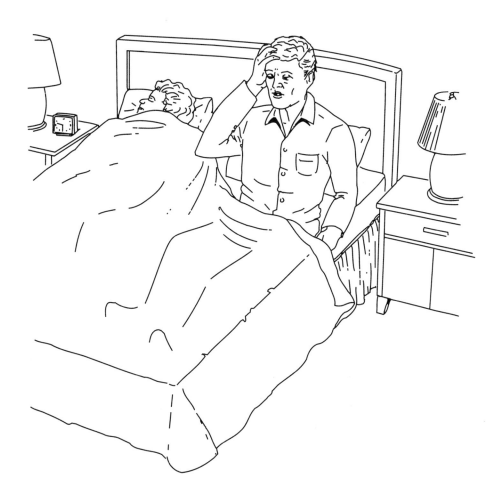

I would have a pounding headache all morning until I
took aspirin to relieve the pain.

California that I needed more exercise, that my problems were stress related, or that I was getting older and my fatigue and depression were normal for my age. But none of these suggestions worked, and the same distressing symptoms persisted year after year.

It was just a coincidence that during a yearly physical examination, I mentioned to my doctor that I was much more tired and irritated during the day, that my snoring had become more intense, and that I was drinking coffee to fight my fatigue. He recommended that I see a sleep specialist, since I had the symptoms of sleep apnea, an ailment that I knew absolutely nothing about.

Because I felt I was getting enough sleep every night, I thought it highly improbable that my years of fatigue and exhaustion resulted from my snoring. But I decided to consult with a sleep specialist at the UCLA Medical Center.

At my initial appointment, within just minutes of completing my physical examination, the doctor unequivocally told me that in all probability I had been suffering from sleep apnea for years without being aware of it. He said the back of my tongue was exceptionally large and my jaw was not in the normal forward position relative to my upper teeth. People with these problems usually have difficulty breathing while they're asleep, resulting in heavy snoring and dangerous sleep apnea. He urged me to have a sleep test to confirm his findings.

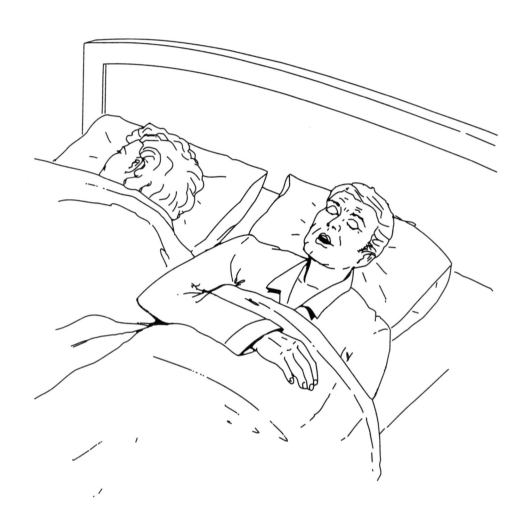

I would stop breathing and gasp for breath
all through the night!

My overnight sleep study was completed on November 22, 1996. I definitely had sleep apnea. It caused me to stop breathing hundreds of times per hour for sometimes as long as two minutes, starving my lungs of precious oxygen and forcing me to wake up repeatedly to gasp for air within minutes of falling asleep. This constant, continuous arousal from sleep night after night was the culprit ruining my life!

It was a miraculous revelation to me to find out that my many years of suffering were related to my heavy snoring and that there was a solution to the problem. For like the vast majority of people, I considered my snoring a fact of life, something that became louder and more intense as I became older.

I have snored for years, and if ever medals were handed out for championship snoring, there is no doubt in my mind or in my family's mind who the unquestioned winner would be. Nobody, but nobody, can beat me in the quality, loudness and intensity of my snoring. My snores can be heard throughout our entire home all during the night. It's irritating and even frightening to anyone unfortunate enough to be in the vicinity of my bedroom.

Anyone sleeping in the same bed with me, or for that matter in the same house, would certainly attest to this fact. Simply ask my wife, my daughter or my son, and they will all tell you in great detail what an annoyance and embarrassment my snoring has been to them over the years.

To save our marriage and sanity, it became necessary many years ago for me to sleep in a separate bedroom, since it was impossible for my wife to get a good night's sleep. My snoring was an irritating problem that caused constant arguing and hard feelings night after night.

Sleeping together was an unpleasant, continuing battle. Every time I would fall asleep and start my annoying snoring and severe tossing and turning, my wife would gently nudge me to interrupt my sleep, hoping that I would turn over to a new position and stop snoring for a few precious minutes so that she could fall asleep before the awful racket started all over again. More often than not, this subtle technique worked without my being aware of it. But when I caught her doing it, I would become infuriated, and insist that I was entitled to sleep and snore if I had to, and that she had absolutely no right to disturb my sleep, since I worked hard all day long, I was the breadwinner of the family, and she would just have to grin and bear the problem. This situation put a serious strain on our marriage for years.

At other times, when the snoring was too intense and annoying to my wife, I would, in an angry huff, grab a blanket and pillow and sleep on the living room sofa just to avoid the arguments and frustration caused by my snoring.

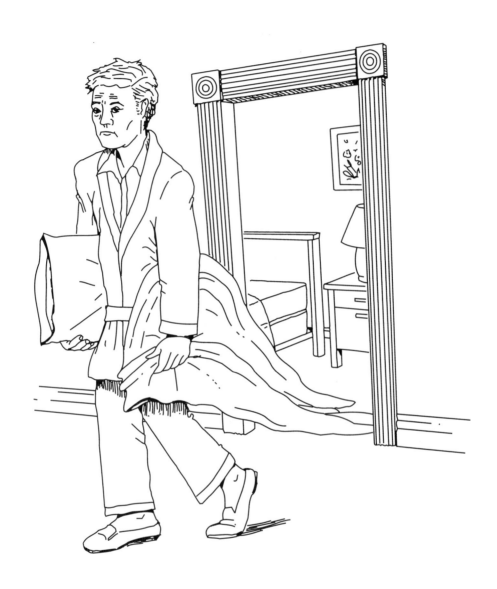

Off to the living room sofa.

My wife still tells our friends of our horrible, embarrassing Caribbean vacation experience. Several years ago, we were staying at a fancy hotel in Puerto Rico that had primitive little cabins right on the beach. It was lovely and very romantic with the moon and the stars and the sound of the ocean. But my nightly snoring was so loud and annoying that the sound carried in the deep silence of the night to other guests in the neighboring cabins, who phoned the front desk to complain about the awful snoring that was keeping them up. We checked out the following morning!

My hope is to warn you about the severe dangers of snoring-related sleep apnea. In approximately 30 minutes of reading time, I want to make you very aware of the causes and consequences of some forms of snoring that can cause death and certainly affect your day-to-day health. I want to alert you to the important warning signs of possible problems, the urgent need for obtaining competent medical advice from the highly qualified, certified sleep disorder specialists, respiratory therapists and sleep disorder dentists that are listed in the appendixes, and above all to urge you to seek immediate help to quickly bring health, vitality and happiness back into your life if you feel you have a sleep-related problem.

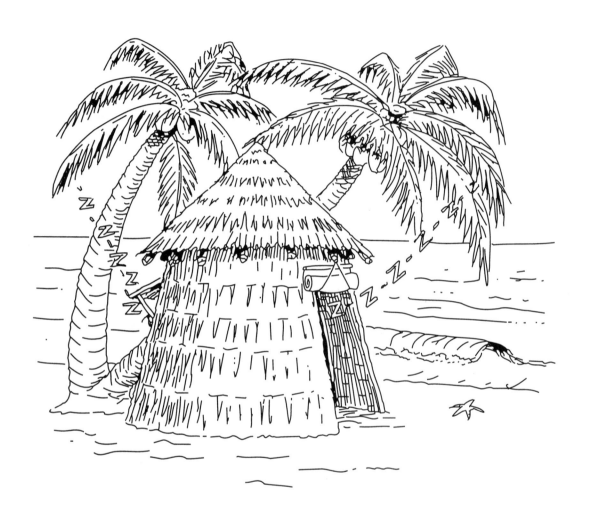

Keep it quiet, your snoring's keeping us up!

He will not suffer me to take my breath . . .
— Job 9.18

Chapter 3

Sleeping, Breathing, Snoring and Sleep Apnea

This year thousands of people throughout the world will die from sleep apnea. Many will die during sleep in the early hours before dawn. The cause of death probably will be listed as a heart attack or "from unknown causes," but in actuality they will have died from an ailment they didn't even know the name of. That ailment is sleep apnea.

It may seem unbelievable, but it is estimated that as many as 30 million Americans of all ages suffer from this unknown killer. However, sleep apnea takes its greatest toll on middle-aged and senior citizens. It is estimated that more than 10 million senior citizens, or approximately 8 million men and 2 million women over the age of 65, in the United States have sleep apnea, and these numbers are increasing daily as the population ages.

To appreciate fully how menacing sleep apnea can be, its effect on your body and the resultant dangers if it's untreated, you must understand the relationship between sleeping, breathing, snoring and, most importantly, sleep apnea.

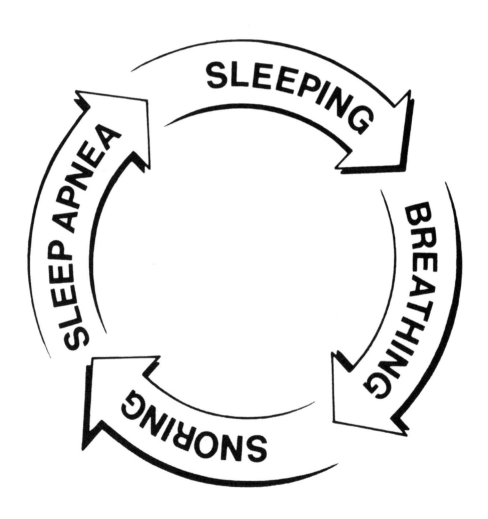

Thou shalt lie down, and thy sleep shall be sweet.

— Proverbs 3.24

Chapter 4

The Mystery of Sleep

We all need a good night's sleep to feel refreshed and adequately energized for our daytime activities. Sleep is far more vital to our health than most people realize. It has a tremendous influence on our overall physical health and our ability to cope with our normal daytime activities. Many of our daily problems, in addition to physical and emotional ailments, can be the result of our inability to get a good night's rest.

Without a good night's sleep, we are irritable, tired all day and unable to work at our maximum efficiency.

Within the last 50 years, the science of sleep has advanced to the unbelievable stage that our sleep can be charted, identified and carefully analyzed. Based on this valuable information, the relationship between sleep and good health has been firmly established.

Experimental tests have been performed in which patients have been deprived of sleep for long periods of time. As a result of this sleep deprivation, psychological problems, mental slowness, lack of alertness and other forms of physical side effects resulted.

Today, with computers and modern technology, it is possible to accurately measure the various stages of sleep, to analyze the quality of sleep, and to discover any problems we may be experiencing during sleep.

When we sleep, we pass through five different levels. Each level is extremely important to our well-being and quality of sleep.

These various levels of sleep are divided into two distinct stages: REM (rapid eye movement) sleep and non-REM sleep. The best sleep requires the proper balance of REM and non-REM sleep. To wake up feeling well rested and physically able to fulfill a normal daytime schedule, it is essential to have not only a sufficient amount of deep REM sleep (about 100 minutes per night) but also the proper proportion of REM and non-REM sleep.

Science has learned that there is a predictable, normal cycle to our sleep pattern.

When we first get into bed, shut off the lights and close our eyes, we enter the first level of non-REM sleep. As we relax, we think about our day's activities, our family, sometimes our problems, and then eventually we doze off into a semihypnotic, relaxing, extremely calm level of sleep. As the minutes go by, we start to sleep more soundly, and our body floats into deeper and deeper levels of non-REM sleep.

During this period of non-REM sleep, significant physical changes take place. The body becomes more and more relaxed and our breathing and brain activity slow down.

About an hour and a half after falling asleep, REM sleep usually takes over from non-REM sleep, with the body cycling between periods of REM and non-REM sleep throughout the night.

REM sleep is very different from non-REM sleep, and it is the deepest, most important stage of the sleep cycle. It is the bewildering dream period that we have all experienced, during which we may have vivid and sometimes weird dreams about our acquaintances, our sexual fantasies or perhaps our childhood, that may or may not be remembered upon awakening. It is essential to reach this stage of sleep nightly if we want to be well rested and healthy.

During critical REM sleep, breathing becomes irregular, alternating between periods of slow and rapid breathing, while the blood circulation within our brain increases. Additionally, our major muscles become paralyzed and, most significantly, our eyes move about rapidly from side to side as if they were watching a tennis match. This "rapid eye movement" gives the REM stage its name.

As the night progresses and the body cycles from one sleep stage to another, the non-REM periods of sleep shorten, while the REM periods increase, especially toward the early morning hours of sleep.

Although we require the proper balance of REM and non-REM sleep, getting a sufficient amount of deep REM sleep is most important for good health and vitality. Unfortunately, many people do not reach this important REM stage of sleep and are troubled with constant fatigue and lack of energy during the day.

Heavy snorers, and especially snorers who are victims of sleep apnea, do not reach this critical REM stage often enough to obtain the benefits of this important level of sleep. The inability to obtain enough REM sleep can have detrimental consequences, causing many undiagnosed serious emotional and physical health problems.

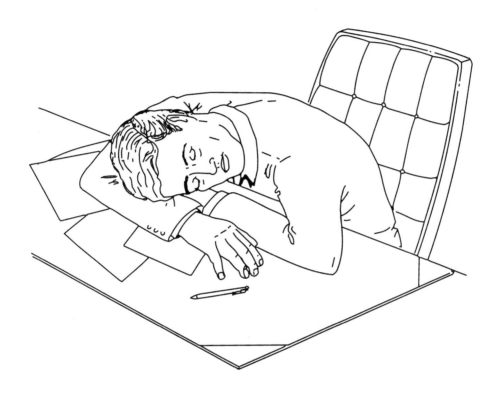

It became increasingly difficult to stay awake during the day.

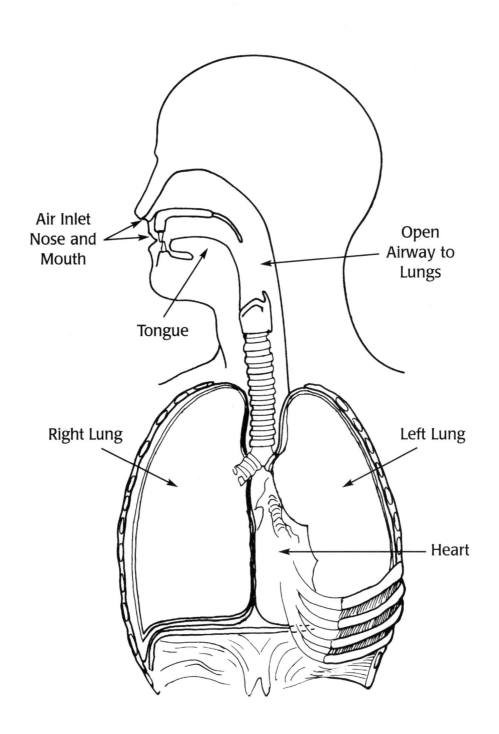

Air Inlet
Nose and
Mouth

Tongue

Right Lung

Open
Airway to
Lungs

Left Lung

Heart

Thou takest away their breath, they die . . .

— Psalms 104.29

Chapter 5

Breathing

Most of us never even think about breathing unless we have a stuffy nose, an allergy or a cold that affects our normal ability to breathe. Breathing is an involuntary physical action we do throughout our life. Although we can hold our breath for a short period of time, we must start breathing again to provide vital oxygen to our brain and body. We take over 20,000 breaths each day to supply our body with oxygen while breathing out carbon dioxide.

Ideally, we should breathe primarily through our nose. As we inhale through our nostrils, the air is filtered, heated and moistened as it starts its path toward our lungs. If we are expending a great deal of energy (perhaps by running or doing other strenuous physical activity), our bodies need more oxygen quickly. So we automatically start breathing through our mouth, since this is a faster and more direct path to get air into our lungs. This action is monitored and controlled by the brain, which constantly checks the amount of gases in the bloodstream. When the brain senses a low level of oxygen and an excess of harmful carbon dioxide in the bloodstream, it sends out an emergency signal to our breathing pump, our diaphragm, which starts pumping harder and faster to furnish more oxygen to our lungs.

Oxygen is the vital fuel our body uses to convert the nutrients in food into energy. In each and every cell of our body, the nutrients combine with the oxygen and burn, producing the energy required for cell growth, vitality and overall good health.

The millions of cells in our body need a continuous supply of oxygen. To furnish this oxygen, we inhale and exhale continuously through our nose and mouth to transport fresh air into our lungs and to discharge the used air, carbon dioxide, out of our body.

The heart is continually pumping fresh blood into our lungs, where the blood combines with pure oxygen. The oxygen-carrying blood then flows through our entire body, delivering to each and every cell fresh fuel and gathering up carbon dioxide, which is transported back into the lungs to be exhaled through our nose and mouth.

This automatic breathing cycle continues over and over again throughout our lifetime and is absolutely essential to human life. Accordingly, it is important that

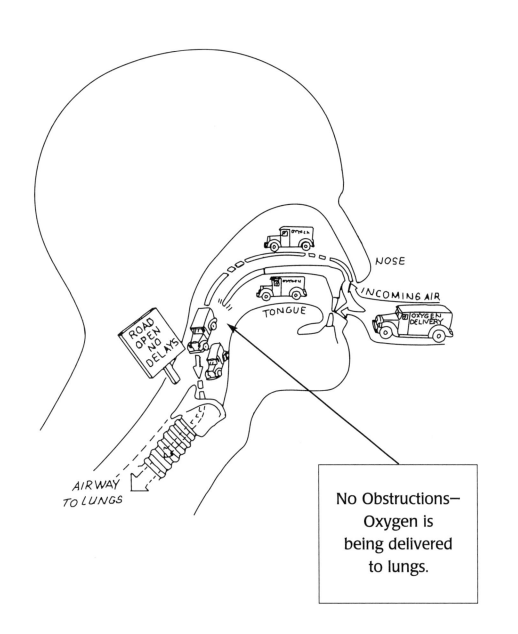

NOSE

INCOMING AIR

OXYGEN DELIVERY

TONGUE

ROAD OPEN NO DELAYS

AIRWAY TO LUNGS

No Obstructions—
Oxygen is
being delivered
to lungs.

there be no obstruction or restriction in our nose, mouth and throat to impede a generous supply of oxygen to our lungs and consequently to our whole body.

For the vast majority of us, breathing during the day is no problem. But during our nighttime sleep, significant changes take place within our body, causing our breathing patterns to change. These new breathing patterns make it much more difficult to breathe and can cause snoring as well as sleep apnea.

There ain't no way to find out why a snorer can't hear himself snore.

— Mark Twain, *Tom Sawyer Abroad*

Chapter 6

Snoring

Imagine driving down a newly paved, two-lane highway. Your drive is smooth, quiet, fast and effortless. Suddenly one lane is closed for repair and traffic is diverted to the other lane. This lane is filled with potholes, road barriers and other road damages, so your drive unexpectedly becomes bumpy, noisy and considerably slower, requiring more physical effort on your part. Basically, this is analogous to the cause of snoring.

During sleep, all the muscles of the body relax, especially in the throat and airway leading to the lungs. This causes the road, or airway, that transports oxygen to the lungs to become narrower, making it extremely difficult to breathe. In addition, the nose may become blocked or congested due to physical abnormalities such as a deviated septum (perhaps caused by a previously broken nose or other old injury) or from an allergy, cold

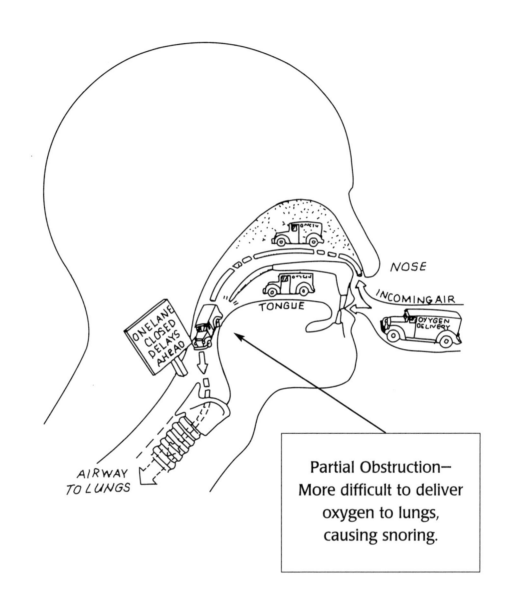

NOSE

INCOMING AIR

OXYGEN DELIVERY

TONGUE

ONE LANE CLOSED DELAYS AHEAD

AIRWAY TO LUNGS

Partial Obstruction—
More difficult to deliver
oxygen to lungs,
causing snoring.

or sinus condition. To complicate matters even more, the tongue may fall backwards toward your throat, especially if you sleep on your back, causing additional narrowing of the airway and further restricting your ability to breathe easily as you attempt to get precious oxygen to your lungs.

All of these partial breathing obstructions caused by muscle relaxation, nasal congestion and tongue movement during sleep produce snoring, which is in actuality a loud vibration, or annoying noise, created in the back part of your throat. The more effort required by your body to breathe during sleep due to these physical obstructions, the louder and more intense will be the snoring level.

Drinking alcohol several hours before bedtime, taking sleeping medications or being overweight will further contribute to the snoring level.

In most instances, nondangerous snoring is a continuous repetition of *snore-snore-snore* sounds without any unusual or frightening nonbreathing or gasping intervals. However, if the cycle consists of snoring, then a period of silence and then a violent gasping for breath, this is a good indicator of problem snoring.

Over 80 million Americans are estimated to snore either nightly or intermittently. For many of these snorers, aside from being annoying, there is only a minimal health risk from snoring. There are safe and effective medical solutions readily available to help a person stop snoring. However, these procedures should only be considered after consultation with qualified medical professionals. For an estimated 30 million snorers in the United States, snoring may be caused by sleep apnea, a far more serious health problem.

To hear a recording of normal snoring as well as dangerous sleep apnea snoring, with a brief explanation of the significant differences between each type, simply phone 1-888-35-SNORE (1-888-357-6673), or on the Internet visit our Web site, snoringcankill.com. Use the password "snore."

Give breath to his nostrils and to his parched throat.
— Unknown, *The Laments*
of Isis and Nepthys

Chapter 7

Sleep Apnea,
The Nighttime Killer

"Apnea: the absence of breathing or
the want of breath."

I learned I had sleep apnea only a few years ago. Until then, I had never heard of this very serious sleep disorder, its dangerous consequences to everyday living and its potential to cause an early death. For these reasons, it's of the utmost importance if you're concerned about excessive snoring to learn the life-threatening facts about sleep apnea and to seek medical advice if you suspect a medical problem.

To easily understand what sleep apnea is and how it affects our health, let's go back to the imaginary two-lane road. In that example, at first the two lanes were open and traffic flowed normally. When one lane was closed and partial obstructions and roadblocks were placed in

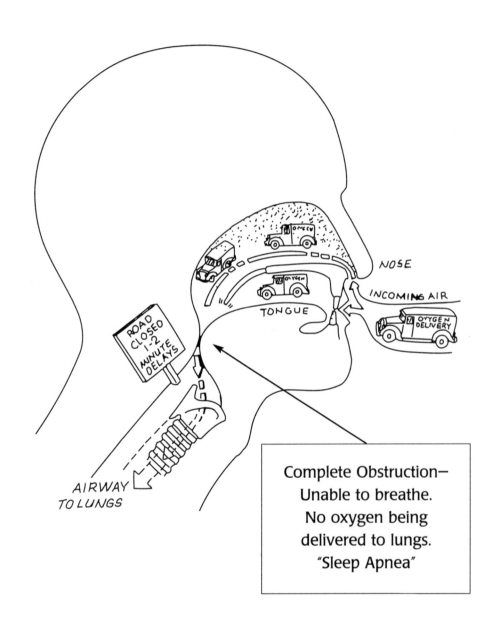

NOSE

INCOMING AIR

OXYGEN
DELIVERY

OXYGEN

TONGUE

ROAD
CLOSED
1-2
MINUTE
DELAYS

AIRWAY
TO LUNGS

Complete Obstruction—
Unable to breathe.
No oxygen being
delivered to lungs.
"Sleep Apnea"

the other lane, traffic continued in just one lane at a slower speed, but eventually everyone arrived at their destination.

Using this same illustration, let's assume that you, the reader, are driving a truck filled with precious oxygen that you must deliver to your own lungs. You are driving along this one-lane obstructed highway, when suddenly you come to an emergency signal, indicating that traffic will be completely stopped for 30 seconds, 60 seconds or perhaps for even as long as two minutes because a fallen tree is blocking the entire road. Imagine also that after you pass this tree, suddenly within just seconds or minutes you reach another obstruction to further delay your trip, once again for 30 seconds, 60 seconds or longer, and that these delays occur over and over and over again, perhaps a hundred or more times each hour of your trip, causing your lungs to be deprived of precious oxygen during each roadway obstruction.

Victims of sleep apnea have a similar problem getting oxygen to their lungs. During sleep, due to physical obstructions such as the muscles in the throat relaxing, nasal congestion or the backward movement of the tongue, the airway becomes totally blocked, making it impossible to breathe and transport needed air to the lungs. This blockage causes a dangerous, deadly, life-threatening lowering of the oxygen level within the body and especially within the brain.

When I was examined to determine what was causing my severe fatigue problems, I was amazed to learn, through a sleep study, of the sequence of violent events taking place nightly during my sleep. I was astounded to discover that as I slept, my throat muscles would relax and my tongue would at the same time flop backwards toward the back of my mouth, completely sealing off the airway to my lungs. My body would be totally and dangerously starved for oxygen for as long as two minutes, and then suddenly an emergency response from my brain would automatically cause me to wake up, gasping for air, and then resume breathing again. Once again, almost immediately I would fall back to sleep, and within a very short time this vicious sleep/no breath/wake up cycle would start again and continue over and over again during the night. I was never aware of or remembered this deadly sleeping and waking up cycle in the morning.

I learned through my sleep study that this was happening hundreds of times per hour and that amazingly I stopped breathing sometimes for as long as two minutes, which would be impossible for me to do while awake!

In addition to learning that I suffered from sleep apnea, I also discovered that some of my nonbreathing episodes were caused by the action of my brain, which simply shut down my breathing mechanism. When the brain is the cause of the apnea, it is called central sleep apnea. The combination of central sleep apnea and apnea caused by a physical obstruction within the airway is called mixed apnea.

Although it is normal and not harmful for most people to stop breathing for a short time during sleep, if within an hour there are 30 or more nonbreathing apnea cycles that last for more than 10 seconds, a person would be diagnosed with sleep apnea.

Depriving the body of oxygen for such long periods of time over and over again, night after night, is the cause of extremely dangerous physical consequences. Elevated blood pressure, heart attacks and strokes, as well as serious emotional and psychotic disorders, can be attributed to sleep apnea, since it deprives precious oxygen to the brain every few seconds or minutes continuously throughout sleep.

In addition to these serious, deadly problems caused by the continuing lack of oxygen to the lungs, sleep apnea creates many other subtle, undiagnosed medical and emotional problems for its victims. These problems are not caused primarily by the lack of oxygen to the body, but by the hundreds and hundreds of waking up, gasping for breath and falling back to sleep cycles that make it almost impossible for a sleep apnea sufferer to reach the REM stage of sleep.

Sleep apnea is a dangerous disorder that requires immediate, competent diagnosis and treatment. There are treatments that can eliminate your snoring to give you a good night's sleep, restore your health and vitality, and eliminate the risk of death from sleep apnea.

If you snore excessively and have any of these symptoms, please consult a sleep specialist:

- High blood pressure
- Excessive daytime sleepiness
- Frequent awakenings during the night
- Frequent trips to the bathroom at night
- Restless sleep
- Falling asleep while driving or at work
- Morning headaches
- Indigestion and/or reflux
- Nausea
- Depression
- Irritable behavior
- Extreme anxiety
- Problems at work
- Impotence
- Dry mouth upon awakening

The beginning of health is sleep.
— **Irish Proverb**

Chapter 8

Sleep Disorder Centers and Your Sleep Study

As mentioned previously, it is unlikely that a doctor can determine if you have a sleep disorder problem, such as sleep apnea, without specialized training and medical certification in this field.

Throughout this book I have suggested over and over again that if you feel that your fatigue and suffering might possibly be due to excessive snoring, you should immediately consult with a sleep specialist. However, with the preponderance of HMOs and other health insurance providers controlling the procedure, in most cases you will first have to discuss your concerns with your primary doctor and review your symptoms and problems. After this discussion, if your doctor concludes that you may possibly have a sleep-related problem, you will be referred to a sleep disorder center.

If, however, you are on Medicare or another health plan that permits you to make your own medical choices, you might want to contact a sleep disorder center directly. Included in Appendix One is a geographic list of sleep disorder centers throughout the United States that have been accredited by the American Sleep Disorders Association. These centers must meet rigid continuing standards, both in state-of-the-art training and sleep test evaluation techniques, for accreditation.

Before being seen by a sleep specialist, you will usually be asked to fill out a form detailing your sleep habits, amount of time slept, your symptoms, and how you felt on each day during a week or more prior to your examination.

When you do visit your sleep specialist, he or she will review and discuss your questionnaire with you and then ask additional, more detailed questions to determine your medical and emotional problems.

A thorough physical examination will then be performed with special emphasis on your nose, throat, tongue, jaw and especially your airway.

Based on this examination and the suspicion that sleep apnea might be the cause of your physical problems, your doctor will recommend that you spend one or two nights at the sleep center for a sleep test to determine if you suffer from sleep apnea.

Usually the first night of the sleep test is to determine if you do have sleep apnea. Just as with an EKG, which is utilized to study your heart, wires will be connected to your body to record and analyze continuously throughout the night the following vital data:

- Brain wave activity—to determine the depth and proportion of REM and non-REM sleep as well as wakefulness and sleep length

- Eye movement

- Vital heart statistics

- Muscle relaxation in jaw, tongue and throat— to determine obstruction

- Leg movement

Additionally, other monitoring devices will be connected to your body to measure your oxygen levels, your inhalation and exhalation levels, and also the degree of muscular difficulty you might experience when you breathe.

Prior to your actual sleep study, you will be prepared for your sleep evaluation by a board-certified sleep technician, who will spend the entire night in an adjacent room monitoring the sleep study equipment. Periodically, the technician will come to your room to make adjustments to the various sensors connected to your body to make certain that you are comfortable and relaxed. If ever during the sleep study you are in distress or need to go to the restroom, the technician is available to disconnect the wiring hookup for your personal convenience.

Based on the data obtained during your first night's sleep study, the sleep doctor will determine if you have sleep apnea and its severity. If you do have sleep apnea, you will be requested to return (usually on the following night) for additional studies to determine the specific treatment to eliminate your sleep apnea.

My sleep was sweet unto me.

— Jeremiah 31.26

Chapter 9

Methods of Treatment

Throughout recorded history, there have been references to sleep apnea and snoring problems. Fortunately for us, the methods of treatment are far more advanced, effective and painless than in years past.

In earlier times, the tongues of sleep apnea sufferers were often stitched to their bottom lip to keep the airway open. Another bizarre procedure involved sewing the tip of the tongue to the front teeth to keep the tongue forward while sleeping. Other painful, and oftentimes brutal, surgical procedures were attempted to cure the problem. Additionally, large, bulky, uncomfortable dental appliances were also utilized that forced the patient's lower jaw forward in order to move the tongue away from the airway.

CPAP

The most significant and beneficial advancement in the treatment of sleep apnea occurred in 1980 in Sydney,

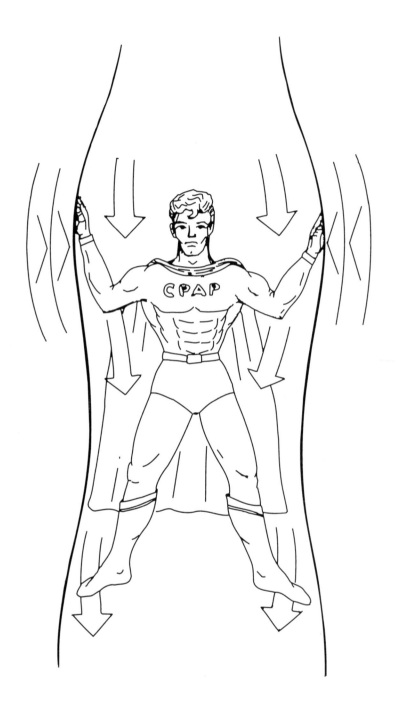

CPAP keeps the airway open so normal breathing
can take place.

Australia, when the brilliant and dedicated sleep researcher, Dr. Colin E. Sullivan, discovered a unique, noninvasive, 100 percent effective technique for eliminating sleep apnea. This technique is recognized throughout the world as state-of-the-art treatment because it has enabled millions of sufferers to obtain a good night's sleep every night without any snoring or gasping for air. They wake up miraculously refreshed and invigorated, thanks to his ingenuity.

Dr. Sullivan's discovery led to the development of small, compact, very efficient machines that blow air through the nostrils into the airway, keeping the passageway from collapsing during sleep so that normal, regular breathing can take place. The air pressure is extremely low, since it is not being used to force air into the lungs, but simply to furnish enough air pressure to keep the airway open.

These are called CPAP (continuous positive air pressure) machines. On the second night of your sleep study, you will use a CPAP machine with a nose mask to see if it will eliminate your sleep apnea and also to determine the proper air settings for your needs. In most instances, during the second night of the sleep study, patients are amazed and delighted at how well they slept and how good they feel in the morning. I certainly did!

If CPAP does work well for you, you will be given a prescription for a machine and a nasal air delivery device and will also be referred to a home health care

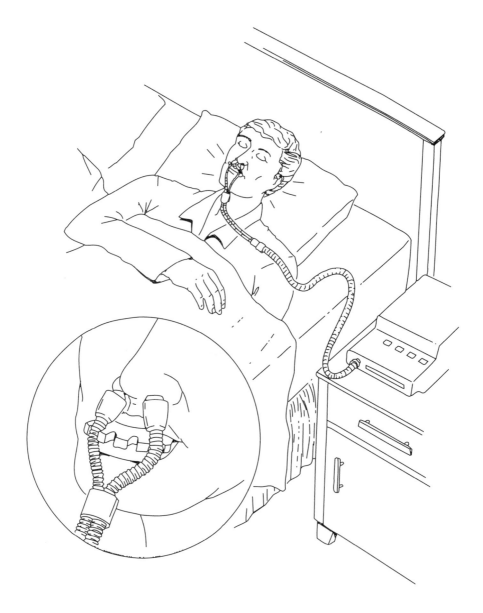

Getting a good night's sleep using a CPAP with a comfortable nasal air delivery device.*

*The illustrated nasal air delivery device is a patented invention of the author. For additional information on this product, contact Caren Publishing Group (310.454.4333).

respiratory therapist to familiarize you with the use of your new equipment, its care and maintenance. Of utmost importance will be the time spent with you by the therapist to ensure that your new nasal air delivery device is the proper size and fit and is comfortable.

The key to your success and health will be the nightly use of your CPAP. Your respiratory therapist will be a vital source of support and advice to make this significant change in your life as easy for you as possible. It is essential that you have a good relationship with your therapist and that you receive proper personalized service to get you through the first difficult months. If you don't, you may be tempted to foolishly discontinue the use of CPAP. This would be unwise and unhealthy since, with help from your respiratory therapist, any problems you may experience can be overcome and you will be provided with a high level of user comfort. DON'T GIVE UP!

If you are not happy with the service, let them know—your life is at stake!

The location of over 600 home health care respiratory therapists who have been recommended by accredited sleep disorder centers throughout the United States are listed in Appendix Two to assist you in locating the best therapist in your area so that you can make this treatment work for you.

Alternative Sleep Apnea Treatments

Dental Devices

During the past several years, tremendous advances have been made by dentists in developing small, very comfortable dental devices that attach to the upper and lower sets of teeth. For many sufferers with mild to moderate sleep apnea who cannot tolerate CPAP, this is an excellent alternative. It is possible to alleviate their disorder by forcing the lower jaw forward with these devices. This action advances the tongue forward, away from the airway, and in many cases opens the airway sufficiently to eliminate the obstruction problem.

Appendix Three contains a list of the Sleep Disorders Dental Society membership. These dentists specialize in the treatment of sleep disorders and work in conjunction with sleep disorder physicians to provide the best solution to sleep apnea problems.

If you are considering the use of a dental device, be sure to first discuss your plans with your sleep doctor and have a sleep test performed using your dental device to be certain it is effective in eliminating your sleep apnea.

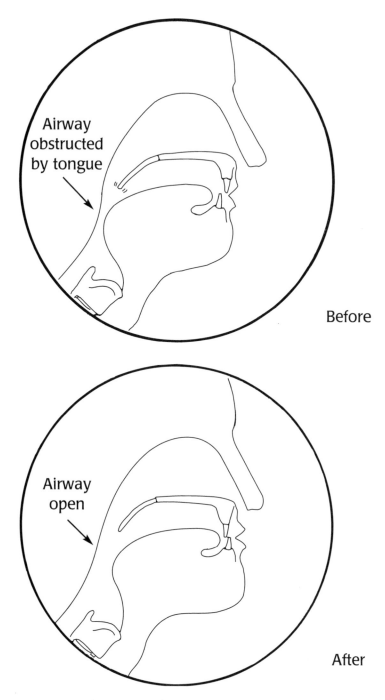

With a dental device (not shown), the jaw and tongue advance forward, opening the airway.

Surgery

In extremely severe cases of sleep apnea that cannot be treated with CPAP or dental devices, surgery may be the best course of treatment, although it is an extreme measure that should only be considered after all other alternatives have been explored. It is a very painful, drastic procedure during which the back of the tongue may be reduced in size, the jaw may be repositioned, and the opening leading into the airway may also be enlarged. Since the success rate is very low, a great deal of deliberation and discussion with your doctors and family should take place before proceeding with this treatment. If, however, you have other life-threatening problems, there may be no alternative to surgery. Consider carefully the risks and benefits of surgery and certainly get a second opinion.

Tracheostomy

Tracheostomy is the treatment of last resort when the patient is in such a weakened state that CPAP or surgery cannot be utilized and no other alternatives exist. A hole is made in the windpipe, below the obstruction, to allow unrestricted inhalation and exhalation. For sleep apnea sufferers, a small cap can be used during the day to seal the opening, and can be easily removed prior to going to sleep. Since the patient is breathing below the blocked section of the airway, healthy breathing is restored. Although it is an extreme measure, it can be 100 percent effective in many cases.

Self-Help Suggestions

In addition to the above treatments, the following will also help to eliminate or reduce the severity of sleep apnea:

- Lose weight to eliminate obesity

- Exercise

- Avoid alcoholic beverages for several hours prior to bedtime

- Discontinue use of sleeping pills and other sleep-inducing drugs (with your doctor's permission)

- Sleep on your side, not on your back

- Use Breathe Right® nasal strips and saline nasal drops for easier breathing through your nose

- Sleep on a wedge or bolster that elevates your head and upper body

- Stop smoking

Sleep is the mystery of life, a wonderful performance of nature.

— **Henri Amiel (1853)**

Chapter 10

Summary

Hopefully, this book has given you some insight and awareness of the possible dangers of nightly snoring. At every opportunity throughout this book, I have suggested over and over again that if you feel there is the *slightest* possibility that you are a victim of this dreadful disorder, you immediately seek competent medical assistance.

This is an extremely serious medical problem that cannot be taken lightly. It can play havoc with your life as well as the lives of your family. It can ruin your career, your marriage and your social life and cause extreme permanent mental and physical problems.

Millions of sleep apnea victims throughout the world have solved their sleeping problems through proper treatment and once again are enjoying lives that are now filled with vim, vigor and vitality.

Please don't hesitate—act now to save your life!!

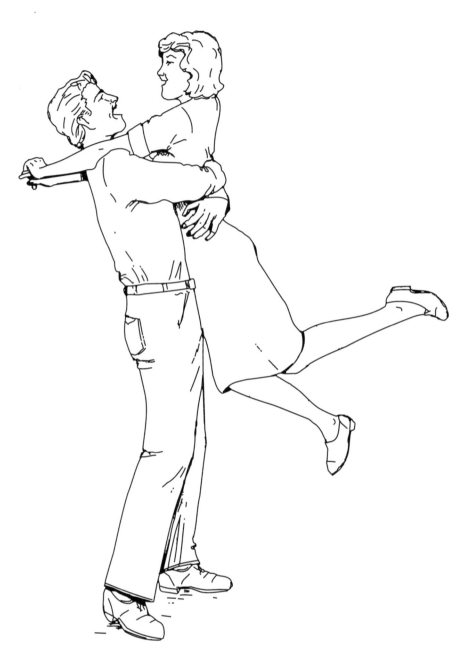

Snoring and sleep apnea can be treated! Act today if you or someone you know has this problem!

Appendixes

American Sleep Disorders Association Accredited Sleep Centers

Sleep disorders include problems with sleeping, staying awake and troublesome behavior during sleep. The American Sleep Disorders Association is dedicated to maintaining high medical standards in the diagnosis and treatment of these difficulties. Following is a listing of sleep disorders centers and laboratories that have been accredited by and maintain membership in the American Sleep Disorders Association. Member Centers provide the diagnosis and treatment of all types of sleep-related disorders, and Member Laboratories (identified with an asterisk) specialize only in sleep-related breathing disorders. The listing is updated on the World Wide Web at http://www.asda.org.

ALABAMA

Sleep-Related Breathing
Disorders Lab*
Athens-Limestone Hosp.
700 W. Market St.
Athens, AL 35612
256-771-REST (7378)

Brookwood Sleep
Disorders Ctr.
Brookwood Medical Ctr.
2010 Brookwood
Med. Ctr. Dr.
Birmingham, AL 35209
205-877-2403

Princeton Sleep/Wake
Disorders Ctr.
Baptist Med. Ctr. Princeton
701 Princeton Ave., S.W.
Birmingham, AL 35211
205-783-7378

Sleep Disorders Ctr. of
Alabama, Inc.
790 Montclair Rd., # 200
Birmingham, AL 35213
205-599-1020

Sleep Disorders Lab*
Carraway Methodist
Med. Ctr.
1600 Carraway Blvd.
Birmingham, AL 35234
205-502-6164

Sleep-Wake Disorders Ctr.
Univ. of Alabama
1713 6th Ave., S.
CPM Bldg., Rm. 270
Birmingham, AL 35233
205-934-7110

Breathing Related Sleep
Disorders Ctr.*
Marshall Med. Ctr. S.
601 A Corley Ave.
Boaz, AL 35957
256-593-1226

Sleep Disorders Ctr.
Cullman Reg. Med. Ctr.
1912 Alabama Hwy. 157
Cullman, AL 35056
256-737-2140

Decatur General Sleep
Disorders Ctr.
1201 7th St., S.E.
Decatur, AL 35601
256-340-2558

Sleep-Wake Disorders Ctr.
Flowers Hosp.
4370 W. Main St.
Dothan, AL 36302
334-793-5000

Thomas Hosp.
Sleep Sevices*
188 Hospital Dr., #201
Fairhope, AL 36532
334-990-1940

ECM Sleep Disorders Lab*
Eliza Coffee Mem. Hosp.
205 Marengo St.
Florence, AL 35631
256-768-9153

Sleep Diagnostics of N.E.
Alabama for Breathing-
Related Disorders
Gadsden Reg. Med. Ctr.*
1007 Goodyear Ave.
Gadsden, AL 35903
256-494-4551

The Crestwood Ctr. for
Sleep Disorders
250 Chateau Dr., # 235
Huntsville, AL 35801
256-880-4710

The Sleep Ctr. at
Huntsville Hosp.
911 Big Cove
Huntsville, AL 35801
256-517-8553

Sleep Disorders Ctr.
Mobile Infirmary Med. Ctr.
P.O. Box 2144
Mobile, AL 36652
334-435-5559

Southeast Reg. Ctr.
for Sleep/Wake Disorders
Springhill Mem. Hosp.
3719 Dauphin St.
Mobile, AL 36608
334-460-5319

USA Knollwood Sleep
Disorders Ctr.
Knollwood Park Hosp.
5644 Girby Rd.
Mobile, AL 36693
334-660-5757

Sleep Disorders Ctr.
Baptist Med. Ctr.
2105 East South Blvd.
Montgomery, AL 36116
334-286-3252

Sleep Disorders Lab*
East Alabama Med. Ctr.
2000 Pepperell Pkwy.
Opelika, AL 36801
334-705-2404

Sleep Disorders Lab*
Helen Keller Hosp.
P.O. Box 610
Sheffield, AL 35660
256-386-4191

Tuscaloosa Clinic Sleep Ctr.
701 University Blvd., E.
Tuscaloosa, AL 35401
205-349-4043

ALASKA

Sleep Disorders Ctr.
Providence Alaska Med. Ctr.
3200 Providence Dr.
Anchorage, AK 99519
907-261-3650

ARIZONA

Samaritan Reg. Sleep
Disorders Program
Thunderbird Samaritan
Med. Ctr.
5555 W. Thunderbird Rd.
Glendale, AZ 85306
602-588-4800

Samaritan Reg. Sleep
Disorders Program
Desert Samaritan Med. Ctr.
1400 South Dobson Rd.
Mesa, AZ 85202
602-835-3684

Samaritan Reg. Sleep
Disorders Program
Good Samaritan
Reg. Med. Ctr.
1111 East McDowell Rd.
Phoenix, AZ 85006
602-239-5815

Sleep Disorders Ctr.
Scottsdale Healthcare Shea
9003 East Shea Blvd.
Scottsdale, AZ 85260
602-860-3200

Sleep Disorders Ctr.
Univ. of Arizona
1501 N. Campbell Ave.
Tucson, AZ 85724
520-694-6112

ARKANSAS

Sleep Disorders Ctr.
Washington Reg. Med. Ctr.
1125 N. College Ave.
Fayetteville, AR 72703
501-713-1272

Pediatric Sleep Disorders
Arkansas Children's Hosp.
800 Marshall St.
Little Rock, AR 72202
501-320-1893

Sleep Disorders Ctr.
Baptist Med. Ctr.
9601 I-630, Exit 7
Little Rock, AR 72205
501-202-1902

CALIFORNIA

Western Med. Centers'
Sleep Disorders Ctr.
1101 S. Anaheim Blvd.
Anaheim, CA 92805
714-491-1159

Sleep Ctr.
Mercy San Juan Hosp.
6401 Coyle Ave., # 109
Carmichael, CA 95608
916-864-5874

Sleep Disorders Institute
St. Jude Med. Ctr.
1915 Sunny Crest Dr.
Fullerton, CA 92835
714-446-7240

Glendale Adventist Med.
Ctr.
Sleep Disorders Ctr.
1509 Wilson Terrace
Glendale, CA 91206
818-409-8323

Pacific Sleep Medicine
Services
La Jolla Ctr.
9834 Genesee Ave., # 328
La Jolla, CA 92037
619-657-0550

Sleep Disorders Ctr.
Grossmont Hosp.
P.O. Box 158
La Mesa, CA 91944
619-644-4488

Loma Linda Sleep
Disorders Ctr.
Loma Linda Univ.
Comm. Med. Ctr.
25333 Barton Rd.
Loma Linda, CA 92354
909-478-6344

Sleep Disorders Ctr.
Long Beach Mem. Med. Ctr.
2801 Atlantic Ave.
Long Beach, CA 90801
562-933-0208

UCLA Sleep Disorders Ctr.
24-221 CHS
Box 957069
Los Angeles, CA 90095
310-206-8005

Los Gatos Clinical
Monitoring Center
Sleep Disorders Ctr.
555 Knowles Dr., # 218
Los Gatos, CA 95032
408-341-2080

Sleep Disorders Ctr.
Hoag Mem. Hosp.
Presbyterian
One Hoag Dr.
Newport Beach, CA 92658
949-760-2070

Sleep Evaluation Ctr.
Northridge Hosp. Med. Ctr.
18300 Roscoe Blvd.
Northridge, CA 91328
818-885-5344

California Ctr. for Sleep
Disorders
3012 Summit St.
5th Floor, South Bldg.
Oakland, CA 94609
510-834-8333

St. Joseph Hosp. Sleep
Disorders Ctr.
1310 W. Stewart Dr., # 403
Orange, CA 92868
714-771-8950

Sleep Disorders Ctr.
UC Irvine
101 City Dr., Route 23
Orange, CA 92868
714-456-5105

Premier Diagnostics, Inc.
1851 Holser Walk, # 210
Oxnard, CA 93030
805-485-2633

Sleep Disorders Ctr.
Huntington Mem. Hosp.
100 W. California Blvd.
Pasadena, CA 91109
626-397-3061

Sleep Disorders Ctr.
Doctors Med. Ctr.
2151 Appian Way
Pinole, CA 94564
510-741-2525

Sleep Disorders Ctr.
Pomona Valley Hosp.
Med. Ctr.
1798 N. Garey Ave.
Pomona, CA 91767
909-865-9587

The Center for Sleep
Apnea*
Redding Med. Ctr.
2701 Eureka Way, # 11
Redding, CA 96001
530-242-6821

Sequoia Sleep Disorders
Ctr.
Sequoia Hosp.
170 Alameda de las Pulgas
Redwood City, CA 94062
650-367-5137

Sutter Sleep Disorders Ctr.
650 Howe Ave., # 910
Sacramento, CA 95825
916-646-3300

UCDMC Sleep Disorders
Ctr.
UCD Med. Ctr.
2315 Stockton Blvd.
Sacramento, CA 95817
916-734-0256

Inland Sleep Ctr.
401 East Highland Ave.
San Bernardino, CA 92404
909-883-8058

Mercy Sleep Disorders Ctr.
Scripps Mercy Hosp.
4077 Fifth Ave.
San Diego, CA 92103
619-260-7378

San Diego Sleep Disorders
Ctr.
1842 Third Ave.
San Diego, CA 92101
619-235-0248

Stanford Health Services
Sleep Clinic
2340 Clay St., # 237
San Francisco, CA 94115
415-923-3336

UCSF/Stanford Sleep
Disorders Ctr. UCSF
1600 Divisadero St.
San Francisco, CA 94115
415-885-7886

The Sleep Disorders Ctr.
of Santa Barbara
2410 Fletcher Ave., # 201
Santa Barbara, CA 93105
805-898-8845

Sleep Disorders Clinic
Stanford Univ. Med. Ctr.
401 Quarry Rd.
Stanford, CA 94305
650-723-6601

Southern California Sleep
Apnea Ctr.*
Lombard Med. Group
2230 Lynn Rd.
Thousand Oaks, CA 91360
805-449-1096

Torrance Mem. Med. Ctr.
Sleep Disorders Ctr.
3330 W. Lomita Blvd.
Torrance, CA 90505
310-517-4617

Sleep Disorders Lab*
Kaweah Delta District
Hosp.
400 W. Mineral King Ave.
Visalia, CA 93291
559-625-7338

West Valley Sleep Disorders
Ctr.
7320 Woodlake Ave., # 140
West Hills, CA 91307
818-715-0096

Sleep Disorders Ctr.
Woodland Mem. Hosp.
1325 Cottonwood St.
Woodland, CA 95695
530-668-2695

COLORADO

National Jewish/Univ. of
Colo. Sleep Ctr.
1400 Jackson St., A200
Denver, CO 80206
303-398-1523

Sleep Disorders Ctr.
St. Luke's Med. Ctr.
1719 E. 19th Ave.
Denver, CO 80218
303-839-6049

Sleep Ctr. of So. Colo.
Parkview Med. Ctr.
400 W. Sixteenth St.
Pueblo, CO 81003
719-584-4659

CONNECTICUT

Danbury Hosp. Sleep
Disorders Ctr.
24 Hospital Ave.
Danbury, CT 06810
203-731-8033

Yale Ctr. for Sleep Disorders
Yale Univ. School of Med.
333 Cedar St.
New Haven, CT 06520
203-737-5556

Gaylord-Wallingford Sleep
Disorders Lab*
Gaylord Hosp.
Gaylord Farms Rd.
Wallingford, CT 06492
203-284-2853

DELAWARE

Sleep Disorders Ctr.
Christiana Care Health
Systems
4755 Ogletown-Stanton Rd.
Newark, DE 19718
302-428-4600

Sleep Disorders Ctr.
Christiana Care Health
Services
Wilmington Hosp.
501 W. 14th St.
Wilmington, DE 19899
302-428-4600

DISTRICT OF COLUMBIA

Sibley Mem. Hosp.
Sleep Disorders Ctr.
5255 Loughboro Rd., N.W.
Washington, DC 20016
202-364-7676

Sleep Disorders Ctr.
Georgetown Univ. Hosp.
3800 Reservoir Rd., N.W.
Washington, DC 20007
202-784-3610

FLORIDA

Boca Raton Sleep Disorders
Ctr.
899 Meadows Rd., # 101
Boca Raton, FL 33486
561-750-9881

Sleep Disorder Lab*
Broward General Med. Ctr.
1600 S. Andrews Ave.
Fort Lauderdale, FL 33316
954-355-5534

Mayo Sleep Disorders Ctr.
Mayo Clinic
4500 San Pablo Rd.
Jacksonville, FL 32224
904-953-7287

Watson Clinic Sleep
Disorders Ctr.
The Watson Clinic, LLP
1600 Lakeland Hills Blvd.
Lakeland, FL 33804
941-680-7627

Atlantic Sleep Disorders Ctr.
1401 S. Apollo Blvd., # A
Melbourne, FL 32901
407-952-5191

Sleep Disorders Ctr.
Miami Children's Hosp.
6125 S.W. 31st St.
Miami, FL 33155
305-669-7136

Sleep Disorders Ctr.
Mt. Sinai Med. Ctr.
4300 Afton Rd.
Miami Beach, FL 33140
305-674-2613

Univ. of Miami School
of Medicine
Sleep Disorders Ctr.
Dept. of Neurology (D4-5)
Miami, FL 33101
305-324-3371

Munroe Reg. Med. Ctr.
Sleep Lab*
131 S.W. 15th St.
Ocala, FL 34473
352-351-7385

Florida Hosp. Sleep
Disorders Ctr.
601 East Rollins Ave.
Orlando, FL 32803
407-897-1558

Orlando Reg. Sleep
Disorders Ctr.
23 W. Copeland Dr.
Orlando, FL 32806
407-649-6869

Health First Sleep
Disorders Ctr.
Palm Bay Comm. Hosp.
1425 Malabar Rd., N.E.
Palm Bay, FL 32907
407-434-8087

Sleep Disorders Ctr.
West Florida Reg. Med. Ctr.
8383 N. Davis Highway
Pensacola, FL 32514
850-494-4850

St. Petersburg Sleep
Disorders Ctr.
2525 Pasadena Ave. S., # S
St. Petersburg, FL 33707
813-360-0853
800-242-3244 (in Florida)

Sleep Disorders Ctr.
Sarasota Mem. Hosp.
1700 S. Tamiami Trail
Sarasota, FL 34239
941-917-2525

Tallahassee Sleep
Disorders Ctr.
1304 Hodges Dr., # B
Tallahassee, FL 32308
800-662-4278 x4 or
850-878-7271

Lab for Sleep-Related
Breathing Disorders*
Univ. Comm. Hosp.
3100 East Fletcher Ave.
Tampa, FL 33613
813-979-7410

GEORGIA

Atlanta Ctr. for Sleep
Disorders
303 Parkway Dr.
Atlanta, GA 30312
404-265-3722

Sleep Disorders Ctr.
Northside Hosp.
5780 Peachtree Dunwoody
Atlanta, GA 30342
404-851-8135

Sleep Disorders Ctr.
of Georgia
5505 Peachtree Dunwoody
Atlanta, GA 30342
404-257-0080

Sleep Disorders Ctr.
Wellstar Cobb Hosp.
3950 Austell Rd.
Austell, GA 30106
770-732-2250

Central Georgia Sleep
Disorders Ctr.
777 Hemlock St., 2nd Fl.
Macon, GA 31202
912-633-7222

Sleep Disorders Ctr.
Wellstar Kennestone Hosp.
677 Church St.
Marietta, GA 30060
770-793-5353

Dept. of Sleep Disorders
Medicine
Candler Hosp.
5353 Reynolds St.
Savannah, GA 31405
912-692-6673

Savannah Sleep Disorders
Ctr.
Saint Joseph's Hosp.
6 St. Joseph's Prof. Plaza
11706 Mercy Blvd.
Savannah, GA 31419
912-927-5141

Sleep Disorders Ctr.
Mem. Health Systems
4700 Waters Ave.
Savannah, GA 31403
912-350-8327

HAWAII

Orchid Isle Sleep
Disorders Lab*
1404 Kilauea Ave.
Hilo, HI 96720
808-935-6105

Pulmonary Sleep
Disorders Ctr.*
Kuakini Med. Ctr.
347 N. Kuakini St.
Honolulu, HI 96817
808-547-9119

Queen's Med. Ctr.
Sleep Lab*
1301 Punchbowl St.
Honolulu, Hl 96813
808-547-4396

Sleep Disorders Ctr.
of the Pacific
Straub Clinic & Hosp.
888 S. King St.
Honolulu, HI 96813
808-522-4448

Orchid Isle Sleep
Disorders Lab*
Waimea Town Plaza
64-1061 Mamalahoa Hwy.
Kamuela, HI 96743
808-885-9681

IDAHO

Idaho Sleep Disorders Ctr.
St. Luke's Reg. Med. Ctr.
190 East Bannock St.
Boise, ID 83712
208-381-2440

Idaho Sleep Disorders Ctr.
Mercy Med. Ctr.
1512 12th Ave.
Nampa, ID 83686
208-463-5820

Idaho Diagnostic
Sleep Lab*
526-C Shoup Ave.
West Twin Falls, ID 83301
208-736-7646

ILLINOIS

Center for Sleep and
Ventilatory Disorders
Univ. of Illinois
1740 W. Taylor St.
Chicago, IL 60612
312-996-7708

Sleep Disorders Ctr.
Northwestern Mem. Hosp.
303 E. Superior Passavant
1044
Chicago, IL 60611
312-908-8120

Sleep Disorders Ctr.
Univ. of Chicago Hospitals
5841 S. Maryland MC2091
Chicago, IL 60637
773-702-1782

Sleep Disorder Service and
Research Ctr.
Rush-Presbyterian-St. Luke's
Med. Ctr.
1653 W. Congress Pkwy.
Chicago, IL 60612
312-942-5440

Sleep Disorders Ctr.
Evanston Hosp.
2650 Ridge Ave.
Evanston, IL 60201
847-570-2567

Sleep Disorders Ctr.
Lutheran General Hosp.
1775 Dempster St.
Park Ridge, IL 60068
847-723-7024

C. Duane Morgan Sleep
Disorders Ctr.
Methodist Med. Ctr.
221 N.E. Glen Oak Ave.
Peoria, IL 61636
309-672-4966

Sleep Disorders Lab*
Rockford Health System
2400 N. Rockton Ave.
Rockford, IL 61103
815-971-5595

SIU School of Medicine
Mem. Med. Ctr.
Sleep Disorders Ctr.
701 N. First
Springfield, IL 62781
217-788-4269

Carle Regional Sleep
Disorders Ctr.
Carle Found. Hosp.
611 W. Park St.
Urbana, IL 61801
217-383-3364

Sleep Disorders Ctr.
Central Du Page Hosp.
25 N. Winfield Rd.
Winfield, IL 60190
630-682-2975

INDIANA

Sleep Disorders Ctr.
St. Francis Hosp. and
Health Centers
1500 Albany St., # I 110
Beech Grove, IN 46107
317-783-8144

St. Mary's Sleep
Disorders Ctr.
St. Mary's Med. Ctr.
3700 Washington Ave.
Evansville, IN 47750
812-485-4960

St. Joseph Sleep
Disorders Ctr.
St. Joseph Med. Ctr.
700 Broadway
Fort Wayne, IN 46802
219-425-3552

Sleep Disorders Ctr.
St. Vincent Hosp. and
Health Services
8401 Harcourt Rd.
Indianapolis, IN 46260
317-338-2152

Sleep/Wake Disorders Ctr.
Comm. Hospitals of
Indianapolis
1500 N. Ritter Ave.
Indianapolis, IN 46219
317-355-4275

Sleep/Wake Disorders Ctr.
Winona Mem. Hosp.
3232 N. Meridian St.
Indianapolis, IN 46208
317-927-2100

Sleep Alertness Ctr.
Lafayette Home Hosp.
2400 South St.
Lafayette, IN 47904
765-447-6811 x 2840

IOWA

Sleep Disorders Ctr.
Mary Greeley Med. Ctr.
1111 Duff Ave.
Ames, IA 50010
515-239-2353

Sleep Disorders Ctr.
Dept. of Neurology
Univ. of Iowa Hospitals and
Clinics
Iowa City, IA 52242
319-356-3813

KANSAS

Sleep Disorders Ctr.
Hays Medical Ctr.
201 E. 7th St.
Hays, KS 67601
785-623-5373

Sleep Disorders Ctr.
St. Francis Hosp. and
Med. Ctr.
1700 S.W. Seventh St.
Topeka, KS 66606
785-295-7900

Sleep Disorders Ctr.
Wesley Med. Ctr.
550 N. Hillside
Wichita, KS 67214
316-688-2663

KENTUCKY

Physicians' Ctr. for
Sleep Disorders
Graves-Gilbert Clinic
201 Park St.
Bowling Green, KY 42102
502-781-5111

Sleep Diagnostics Lab*
Greenview Reg. Hosp.
1801 Ashley Cir.
Bowling Green, KY 42101
502-793-2175

Sleep Disorders Ctr.
St. Luke Hosp. West
7380 Turfway Rd.
Florence, KY 41042
606-525-5347

The Sleep Disorder Ctr. of
St. Luke Hosp.
85 N. Grand Ave.
Fort Thomas, KY 41075
606-572-3535

Sleep Apnea Ctr.*
Jennie Stuart Med. Ctr.
320 W. 18th St.
Hopkinsville, KY 42240
502-887-0410

Sleep Apnea Ctr.*
Samaritan Hosp.
310 S. Limestone
Lexington, KY 40508
606-252-6612 x7331

Sleep Disorders Ctr.
St. Joseph's Hosp.
One St. Joseph Dr.
Lexington, KY 40504
606-278-0444

Caritas Sleep Apnea Ctr.*
Caritas Med. Ctr.
1850 Bluegrass Ave.
Louisville, KY 40215
502-361-6555

Sleep Disorders Ctr.
Audubon Hosp.
One Audubon Plaza Dr.
Louisville, KY 40217
502-636-7459

Sleep Disorders Ctr.
Univ. of Louisville Hosp.
530 S. Jackson St.
Louisville, KY 40202
502-562-3792

Sleep Medicine Specialists
1169 Eastern Pkwy., # 3357
Louisville, KY 40217
502-454-0755

Regional Med. Ctr. Lab for
Sleep-Related Breathing
Disorders*
900 Hospital Dr.
Madisonville, KY 42431
502-825-5918

Diller Regional Sleep
Disorders Ctr.
Lourdes Hosp.
1530 Lone Oak Rd.
Paducah, KY 42001
502-444-2660

Breathing Disorders Sleep
Lab*
Pikeville Methodist Hosp.
911 S. Bypass Rd.
Pikeville, KY 41501
606-437-3989

P.A.C. Sleep Disorders Lab*
Pattie A. Clay Hosp.
801 Eastern Bypass
Richmond, KY 40475
606-625-3334

The Med. Ctr. Sleep Lab*
456 Burnley Rd.
Scottsville KY 42164
502-622-2865

LOUISIANA

Lourdes Sleep Disorders
Ctr.
Our Lady of Lourdes Reg.
Med. Ctr.
611 St. Landry
Lafayette, LA 70506
318-289-2858

Mem. Med. Ctr. Sleep
Disorders Ctr.
2700 Napoleon Ave.
New Orleans, LA 70115
504-896-5652

Tulane Sleep Disorders Ctr.
1415 Tulane Ave.
New Orleans, LA 70112
504-588-5231

LSU Sleep Disorders Ctr.
Louisiana State Univ.
Med. Ctr.
P.O. Box 33932
Shreveport, LA 71130
318-675-5365

Neurology & Sleep Clinic
2205 E. 70th St.
Shreveport, LA 71105
318-797-1585

NSRMC Sleep
Disorders Ctr.
No. Shore Reg. Med. Ctr.
100 Med. Ctr. Dr.
Slidell, LA 70461
504-646-5711

MAINE

St. Mary's Sleep Disorders
Lab*
St. Mary's Reg. Med. Ctr.
97 Campus Ave.
Lewiston, ME 04240
207-777-8959

Maine Institute for Sleep
Breathing Disorders*
930 Congress St.
Portland, ME 04102
207-871-4535

MARYLAND

The Johns Hopkins Sleep
Disorders Ctr.
Asthma and Allergy Bldg.
5501 Hopkins Bayview Cir.
Baltimore, MD 21224
410-550-0571

Maryland Sleep Disorders
Ctr.
Greater Baltimore Med. Ctr.
6701 N. Charles St., # 4140
Baltimore, MD 21204
410-494-9773

Frederick Sleep Disorders
Ctr.
Frederick Mem. Hosp.
400 W. Seventh St.
Frederick, MD 21701
301-698-3802

Sleep-Breathing Disorders
Ctr. of Hagerstown*
12821 Oak Hill Ave.
Hagerstown, MD 21742
301-733-5971

Shady Grove Sleep
Disorders Ctr.
14915 Broschart Rd., # 102
Rockville, MD 20850
301-251-5905

Washington Adventist Sleep
Disorders Ctr.
7525 Carroll Ave.
Takoma Park, MD 20912
301-891-2594

MASSACHUSETTS

Sleep Disorders Ctr.
Beth Israel Deaconess Med.
Ctr.
330 Brookline Ave., KS430
Boston, MA 02215
617-667-3237

Sleep Disorders Ctr.
Lahey Clinic
41 Mail Rd.
Burlington, MA 01805
781-744-8251

Sleep Disorders Institute
of Central New England
St. Vincent Hosp.
25 Winthrop St.
Worcester, MA 01604
508-798-6212

MICHIGAN

Sleep Disorders Ctr.
St. Joseph Mercy Hosp.
P.O. Box 995
Ann Arbor, MI 48106
734-712-4651

Sleep Disorders Ctr.
Univ. of Michigan Hospitals
1500 East Med. Ctr. Dr.
Ann Arbor, MI 48109
734-936-9068

Sleep Disorders Clinic
Bay Med. Ctr.
1900 Columbus Ave.
Bay City, MI 48708
517-894-3332

Harper Hosp. Sleep
Disorders Ctr.
4160 John R St., # 400
Detroit, MI 48201
313-745-9009

Sinai Sleep Ctr.
DMC Sinai Hosp.
6767 W. Outer Dr.
Detroit, MI 48235
313-493-5148

Sleep/Wake Disorders Lab
VA Med. Ctr.
4646 John R St.
Detroit, MI 48201
313-576-3663

West Michigan Sleep
Disorders Ctr.
Butterworth Hosp.
100 Michigan St., N.E.
Grand Rapids, MI 49503
616-391-3759

Sleep Disorders Ctr.
Borgess Med. Ctr.
1521 Gull Rd.
Kalamazoo, MI 49001
616-226-7081

Ingham Regional Med. Ctr.
Sleep/Wake Ctr.
2025 S. Washington Ave.
Lansing, MI 48910
517-372-6444

Sparrow Sleep Ctr.
Sparrow Hosp.
1215 E. Michigan Ave.
Lansing, MI 48909
517-364-5370

Sleep & Respiratory
Associates of Michigan
28200 Franklin Rd.
Southfield, MI 48034
248-350-2722

Munson Sleep Disorders
Ctr.
Munson Med. Ctr.
1105 Sixth St., MPB, # 307
Traverse City, MI 49684
800-358-9641 or
616-935-6600

Sleep Disorders Institute
44199 Dequindre, # 311
Troy, MI 48098
248-879-0707

MINNESOTA

Duluth Regional Sleep
Disorders Ctr.
St. Mary's Duluth Clinic
Health System
407 E. Third St.
Duluth, MN 55805
218-726-4692

Fairview Sleep Ctr.
Fairview Southdale Hosp.
6401 France Ave., S.
Edina, MN 55435
612-924-5053

Minnesota Regional Sleep
Disorders Ctr.
#867B Hennepin County
Med. Ctr.
701 Park Ave., S.
Minneapolis, MN 55415
612-347-6288

Sleep Disorders Ctr.
Abbott N.W. Hosp.
800 E. 28th St.
Minneapolis, MN 55407
612-863-4516

Mayo Sleep Disorders Ctr.
Mayo Clinic
200 First St., S.W.
Rochester, MN 55905
507-266-8900

Sleep Disorders Ctr.
Methodist Hosp.
6500 Excelsior Blvd.
St. Louis Park, MN 55426
612-993-6083

St. Joseph's Sleep
Diagnostic Ctr.
St. Joseph's Hosp.
69 W. Exchange St.
St. Paul, MN 55102
612-232-3682

MISSISSIPPI

Sleep Disorders Ctr.
Mem. Hosp.
P.O. Box 1810
Gulfport, MS 39501
601-865-3152

Sleep Disorders Ctr.
Forrest General Hosp.
6051 Highway 49
Hattiesburg, MS 39404
601-288-4790

Sleep Disorders Ctr.
Univ. of Miss. Med. Ctr.
2500 N. State St.
Jackson, MS 39216
601-984-4820

MISSOURI

Unity Sleep Medicine
and Research Ctr.
St. Luke's Hosp.
232 S. Woods Mill Rd.
Chesterfield, MO 63017
314-205-6030

Univ. of Missouri Sleep
Disorders Ctr.
M-741 Neurology
Univ. Hosp. and Clinics
One Hospital Dr.
Columbia, MO 65212
573-884-SLEEP

Sleep Disorders Ctr.
Research Med. Ctr.
2316 E. Meyer Blvd.
Kansas City, MO 64132
816-276-4334

Sleep Disorders Ctr.
St. Luke's Hosp.
4400 Wornall Rd.
Kansas City, MO 64111
816-932-3207

Sleep Disorders &
Research Ctr.
Deaconess Med. Ctr.
6150 Oakland Ave.
St. Louis, MO 63139
314-768-3100

Sleep/Wake Disorders Ctr.
The Health Services Div. of
Saint Louis Univ.
1221 S. Grand Blvd.
St. Louis, MO 63104
314-577-8705

Cox Regional Sleep
Disorders Ctr.
3800 S. National Ave.
Springfield, MO 65807
417-269-5575

St. John's Sleep Disorders
Ctr.
St. John's Reg. Health Ctr.
1235 E. Cherokee
Springfield, MO 65804
417-885-5464

MONTANA

The Sleep Ctr. at St. Vincent
Hosp.
1233 N. 30th St.
Billings, MT 59101
406-238-6815

Sleep Disorders Ctr.
Deaconess Billings Clinic
2800 Tenth Ave., N.
Billings, MT 59107
406-657-4075

NEBRASKA

Adult and Pediatric Sleep-
Related Breathing Disorders
Lab*
Bryan LGH Mem. Ctr. East
1600 S. 48th St.
Lincoln, NE 68506
402-483-3950

Great Plains Regional Sleep
Physiology Ctr.
Bryan LGH Med. Ctr. West
2300 S. 16th St.
Lincoln, NE 68502
402-473-5338

Sleep Disorders Ctr.
Methodist/Richard Young
Hosp.
2566 St. Mary's Ave.
Omaha, NE 68105
402-354-6305

Sleep Disorders Ctr.
Nebraska Health System

4350 Dewey Ave.
Omaha, NE 68105
402-552-2286

NEVADA

Mountain Med. Sleep
Disorders Ctr.
Mountain Med. Assoc., Inc.
710 W. Washington St.
Carson City, NV 89703
775-882-2106

The Sleep Clinic of Nevada
1012 East Sahara Ave.
Las Vegas, NV 89104
702-893-0020

Washoe Sleep Disorders Ctr.
and Sleep Lab
Washoe Professional Bldg.
75 Pringle Way, # 701
Reno, NV 89502
775-328-4700 or
800-JETLAGG

NEW HAMPSHIRE

Sleep Disorders Ctr.
Dartmouth-Hitchcock
Med. Ctr.
One Med. Ctr. Dr.
Lebanon, NH 03756
603-650-7534

Ctr. for Sleep Evaluation
Catholic Med. Ctr.
100 McGregor St.
Manchester, NH 03102
603-663-6680

NEW JERSEY

SleepCare Ctr. of
Cherry Hill
457 Haddonfield Rd., # 520
Cherry Hill, NJ 08002
800-753-3779

Sleep Lab Institute for
Sleep/Wake Disorders
Hackensack Univ. Med. Ctr.
30 Prospect Ave.
Hackensack, NJ 07601
201-996-2992

Morristown Sleep
Disorder Ctr.
Morristown Mem. Hosp.
95 Mount Kemble Ave.
Morristown, NJ 07962
973-971-4567

SleepCare Mem. Hosp. of
Burlington County
175 Madison Ave.
Mount Holly, NJ 08060
800-753-3779

Sleep Disorders Ctr.
Newark Beth Israel Med.
Ctr.
201 Lyons Ave.
Newark, NJ 07112
973-926-6668

Comprehensive Sleep
Disorders Ctr.
Robert Wood Johnson
Univ. Hosp./ UMDNJ
1 Robert Wood
Johnson Pl.
New Brunswick, NJ 08903
732-937-8683

Sleep Disorders Ctr.
Capital Health System at
Mercer
446 Bellevue Ave.
Trenton, NJ 08607
609-394-4167

Snoring and Sleep Apnea
Ctr.*
Helene Fuld Med. Ctr.
750 Brunswick Ave.
Trenton, NJ 08638
609-278-6990

Sleep Disorders Ctr. of
New Jersey
2253 South Ave., # 7
Westfield, NJ 07090
908-789-4244

NEW MEXICO

Lovelace Sleep Disorders
Ctr.
Lovelace Health Systems
2929 Coors Blvd., N.W.
Albuquerque, NM 87120
505-839-2369

Univ. Hosp. Sleep
Disorders Ctr.
4775 Indian School Rd.,
N.E., # 307
Albuquerque, NM 87110
505-272-6101

NEW YORK

Capital Region Sleep/Wake
Disorders Ctr.
St. Peter's Hosp.
West Plaza #1
Washington Ave. Ext.
Albany, NY 12205
518-436-9253

Sleep/Wake Disorders Ctr.
Montefiore Med. Ctr.
111 E. 210th St.
Bronx, NY 10467
718-920-4841

Bassett Healthcare Sleep
Disorders Ctr.
One Atwell Rd.
Cooperstown, NY 13326
607-547-6979

St. Joseph's Hosp. Sleep
Disorders Ctr.
555 E. Market St.
Elmira, NY 14902
607-737-7008

Sleep Disorders Ctr.
Winthrop-Univ. Hosp.
222 Station Plaza, N.
Mineola, NY 11501
516-663-3907

Sleep-Wake Disorders Ctr.
Long Island Jewish Med.
Ctr.
270-05 76th Ave.
New Hyde Park, NY 11042
718-470-7058

The Sleep Disorders Ctr.
Columbia-Presbyterian
Med. Ctr.
161 Fort Washington Ave.
New York, NY 10032
212-305-1860

Sleep Disorders Institute
1090 Amsterdam Ave.
New York, NY 10025
212-523-1700

Sleep-Wake Disorders Ctr.
New York Hosp., Cornell
Manhattan Campus
520 E. 70th St.
New York, NY 10021
914-997-5751

Sleep Disorders Ctr. of
Rochester
2110 Clinton Ave., S.
Rochester, NY 14618
716-442-4141

Sleep Disorders Ctr.
SUNY at Stony Brook
Univ. Hosp. MR 120 A
Stony Brook, NY 11794
516-444-2916

Sleep Ctr. Comm. Gen.
Hosp.
Broad Rd.
Syracuse, NY 13215
315-492-5877

The Sleep Lab*
St. Joseph's Hosp.
Health Ctr.
945 East Genesee St., # 300
Syracuse, NY 13210
315-475-3379

The Mohawk Valley Sleep
Disorders Ctr.
St. Elizabeth Med. Ctr.
2209 Genesee St.
Utica, NY 13501
315-734-3484

The Sleep Disorders Ctr.
White Plains Columbia-
Presbyterian Med. Ctr.
185 Maple Ave.
White Plains, NY 10601
914-948-0400

Sleep-Wake Disorders Ctr.
New York Hosp.-Cornell
Med. Ctr.
21 Bloomingdale Rd.
White Plains, NY 10605
914-997-5751

NORTH CAROLINA

Sleep Medicine Ctr. of
WNC
1091 Hendersonville Rd.
Asheville, NC 28803
704-277-7533

Western Carolina Sleep Ctr.
Mission/St. Joseph's
Health System
445 Biltmore Ave., # 404
Asheville, NC 28801
828-258-6701

Carolinas Sleep Services
Mercy Hosp. S.
16028 Park Rd.
Charlotte, NC 28210
704-543-2213

Carolinas Sleep Services
Univ. Hosp.
8800 N. Tyron St.
Charlotte, NC 28256
704-548-5855

Sleep Disorders Ctr.
Moses Cone Health System
1200 N. Elm St.
Greensboro, NC 27401
336-832-7406

Sleep Medicine Ctr. of
Salisbury
911 W. Henderson St., # L30
Salisbury, NC 28144
704-637-1533

Sleep Disorders Ctr.
N. Carolina Baptist Hosp.
Wake Forest Univ. School
of Medicine
Med. Ctr. Blvd.
Winston-Salem, NC 27157
336-716-5288

Summit Sleep Disorders
Ctr.
160 Charlois Blvd.
Winston-Salem, NC 27103
336-765-9431

NORTH DAKOTA

No Accredited Member
Centers

OHIO

Cincinnati Reg. Sleep Ctrs.
2123 Auburn Ave., #322
Cincinnati, OH 45219
513-721-4680

Sleep Disorders Ctr. of
Greater Cincinnati
TriHealth Hospitals
619 Oak St.
Cincinnati, OH 45206
513-569-6320

The Tri-State Sleep
Disorders Ctr.
1275 East Kemper Rd.
Cincinnati, OH 45246
513-671-3101

PMA Cardiopulmonary
Sleep Lab*
Pulmonary Medicine
Assoc., Inc.
15805 Puritas Ave.
Cleveland, OH 44135
216-267-5933

Sleep Disorders Ctr.
Cleveland Clinic Found.
9500 Euclid Ave., Desk S-51
Cleveland, OH 44195
216-444-2165

Univ. Hospitals Sleep Ctr.
Univ. Hospitals of
Cleveland, Dept. of
Neurology
11100 Euclid Ave.
Cleveland, OH 44106
216-844-1301

Sleep Disorders Ctr.
OSU Med. Ctr.
Rhodes Hall, S1039
410 W. 10th Ave.
Columbus, OH 43210-1228
614-293-8296

The Ctr. for Sleep & Wake
Disorders
Miami Valley Hosp.
One Wyoming St., # G-200
Dayton, OH 45409
937-208-2515

Sleep Disorders Ctr.
Good Samaritan Hosp.
2222 Philadelphia Dr.
Dayton, OH 45406
937-276-8307

Ohio Sleep Medicine and
Neuroscience Institute
4975 Bradenton Ave.
Dublin, OH 43017
614-766-0773

Sleep Disorders Ctr.
Kettering Med. Ctr.
3535 Southern Blvd.
Kettering, OH 45429
937-296-7805

Ohio Sleep Disorders Ctr.
150 Springside Dr.
Montrose, OH 44333
330-670-1290

N.W. Ohio Sleep Disorders
Ctr.
The Toledo Hosp.
Harris-McIntosh Tower
2142 N. Cove Blvd.
Toledo, OH 43606
419-471-5629

Sleep Disorders Ctr.
Genesis Health Care System
Good Samaritan Med. Ctr.
800 Forest Ave.
Zanesville, OH 43701
740-454-5855

OKLAHOMA

Sleep Disorders Ctr. of
Oklahoma
Integris Health
4401 S. Western Ave.
Oklahoma City, OK 73109
405-636-7700

OREGON

Sleep Disorders Ctr.
Sacred Heart Med. Ctr.
1255 Hilyard St.
Eugene, OR 97440
503-686-7224

Sleep Disorders Ctr.
Rogue Valley Med. Ctr.
2825 East Barnett Rd.
Medford, OR 97504
541-608-4320

Legacy Good Samaritan
Sleep Disorders Ctr.
Neurology, T-302
1015 Northwest 22nd Ave.
Portland, OR 97210
503-413-7540

Pacific N.W. Sleep/Wake
Disorders Program
1849 N.W. Kearney, # 202
Portland, OR 97209
503-228-4414

Sleep Disorders Lab*
Providence Portland
Med. Ctr.
4805 N.E. Glisan St.
Portland, OR 97213
503-215-6552

Salem Hosp. Sleep
Disorders Ctr.
Salem Hosp.
665 Winter St., S.E.
Salem, OR 97309
503-370-5170

PENNSYLVANIA

Sleep Disorders Ctr.
Abington Mem. Hosp.
1200 Old York Rd.
Abington, PA 19001
215-576-2226

Sacred Heart Sleep
Disorders Ctr.
Sacred Heart Hosp.
421 Chew St.
Allentown, PA 18102
610-776-5333

Sleep Disorders Ctr.
Lower Bucks Hosp.
501 Bath Rd.
Bristol, PA 19007
215-785-9752

Penn Ctr. for Sleep
Disorders
800 W. State St.
Doylestown, PA 18901
215-345-5003

Sleep Disorders Ctr. of
Lancaster
Lancaster Gen. Hosp.
555 N. Duke St.
Lancaster, PA 17604
717-290-5910

Saint Mary Sleep/Wake
Disorder Ctr.
Langhorne-Newtown Rd.
Langhorne, PA 19047
215-741-6744

Sleep Medicine Services at
Paoli Mem. Hosp.
255 W. Lancaster Ave.
Paoli, PA 19301
610-645-3400

Penn Ctr. for Sleep
Disorders
Univ. of Penn. Med. Ctr.
3400 Spruce St.
Philadelphia, PA 19104
215-662-7772

Pennsylvania Hosp. Sleep
Disorders Ctr.
Eighth and Spruce Streets
Philadelphia, PA 19107
215-829-7079

Sleep Disorders Ctr.,
Dept. of Neurology
MCP-Hahnemann School
of Medicine
3200 Henry Ave.
Philadelphia, PA 19129
215-842-4250

Sleep Disorders Ctr.
Thomas Jefferson Univ.
1015 Walnut St., # 319
Philadelphia, PA 19107
215-955-6175

Temple Sleep Disorders Ctr.
Temple Univ. Hosp.
3401 N. Broad St.
Philadelphia, PA 19140
215-707-8163

Pulmonary Sleep
Evaluation Lab*
Montefiore Univ. Hosp.
3459 Fifth Ave., S639
Pittsburgh, PA 15213
412-692-2880

Sleep and Chronobiology
Ctr.
Western Psychiatric Inst. &
Clinic
3811 O'Hara St.
Pittsburgh, PA 15213
412-624-2246

Crozer Sleep Disorders Ctr.
at Taylor Hosp.
175 East Chester Pike
Ridley Park, PA 19078
610-595-6272

Sleep Disorders Ctr.
Comm. Med. Ctr.
1822 Mulberry St.
Scranton, PA 18510
717-969-8931

Sleep Disorders Ctr.
Mercy Hosp.
25 Church St.
Wilkes-Barre, PA 18765
717-826-3410

Sleep Disorders Ctr.
Lankenau Hosp.
100 Lancaster Ave.
Wynnewood, PA 19096
610-645-3400

RHODE ISLAND

No Accredited Member
Centers

SOUTH CAROLINA

Roper Sleep/Wake
Disorders Ctr.
Roper Hosp.
316 Calhoun St.
Charleston, SC 29401
843-724-2246

Sleep Disorders Ctr.
S.C. Baptist Med. Ctr.
Taylor at Marion Sts.
Columbia, SC 29220
803-771-5847 or
800-368-1971

Southeast Regional Sleep
Disorders Ctr. Easley
200 Fleetwood Dr.
Easley, SC 29640
864-855-7200

Sleep Disorders Ctr.
Greenville Mem. Hosp.
701 Grove Rd.
Greenville, SC 29605
864-455-8916

Southeast Reg. Sleep
Disorders Ctr.
3900 Pelham Rd.
Greenville, SC 29615
864-627-5337

Carolinas Sleep Services
1665 Herlong Court, # B
Rock Hill, SC 29732
803-817-1915

Sleep Disorders Ctr.
Spartanburg Regional
Med. Ctr.
101 E. Wood St.
Spartanburg, SC 29303
864-560-6904

SOUTH DAKOTA

The Sleep Ctr.
Rapid City Regional Hosp.
353 Fairmont Blvd.
Rapid City, SD 57709
605-341-8037

Sleep Disorders Ctr.
Sioux Valley Hosp.
1100 South Euclid
Sioux Falls, SD 57117
605-333-6302

TENNESSEE

Summit Ctr. for Sleep
Related Breathing
Disorders*
Columbia-Summit
Med. Ctr.
5655 Frist Blvd.
Hermitage, TN 37076
615-316-3495

Sleep Disorders Lab*
Regional Hosp. of Jackson
367 Hosp. Blvd.
Jackson, TN 38303
901-661-2148

Sleep Disorders Ctr.
Ft. Sanders Regional
Med. Ctr.
1901 W. Clinch Ave.
Knoxville, TN 37916
423-541-1375

Sleep Disorders Ctr.
St. Mary's Med. Ctr.
900 East Oak Hill Ave.
Knoxville, TN 37917
423-545-6746

BMH Sleep Disorders Ctr.
Baptist Mem. Hosp.
899 Madison Ave.
Memphis, TN 38146
901-227-5337

Sleep Disorders Ctr.
Methodist Hospitals of
Memphis
1265 Union Ave.
Memphis, TN 38104
901-726-REST

Sleep Disorders Ctr.
Middle Tenn. Med. Ctr.
400 N. Highland Ave.
Murfreesboro, TN 37130
615-849-4811

Baptist Sleep Ctr.
Baptist Hosp.
2000 Church St.
Nashville, TN 37236
615-329-6306

Sleep Disorders Ctr.
Centennial Med. Ctr.
2300 Patterson St.
Nashville, TN 37203
615-342-1670

Sleep Disorders Ctr.
Saint Thomas Hosp.
P.O. Box 380
Nashville, TN 37202
615-222-2068

TEXAS

NWTH Sleep Disorders Ctr.
Northwest Texas Hosp.
P.O. Box 1110
Amarillo, TX 79175
806-354-1954

Sleep Disorders Ctr. for
Children
Children's Med. Ctr.
1935 Motor St.
Dallas, TX 75235
214-640-2793

Sleep Medicine Institute
Presbyterian Hosp.
8200 Walnut Hill Lane
Dallas, TX 75231
214-750-7776

Sleep Disorders Ctr.
Columbia Med. Ctr. West
1801 N. Oregon
El Paso, TX 79902
915-521-1257

Sleep Disorders Ctr.
Columbia Med. Ctr.
10301 Gateway West
El Paso, TX 79925
915-594-5882

Sleep Disorders Ctr.
Providence Mem. Hosp.
2001 N. Oregon
El Paso, TX 79902
915-577-6152

Sleep Consultants, Inc.
1521 Cooper St.
Fort Worth, TX 76104
817-332-7433

The Sleep Ctr.
Spring Branch Med. Ctr.
8850 Long Point Rd.
Houston, TX 77055
713-984-3519

Sleep Disorders Ctr.
Dept. of Psychiatry
Baylor College of Medicine
and VA Med. Ctr.
One Baylor Plaza
Houston, TX 77030
713-798-4886

Sleep Disorders Ctr.
Scott and White Clinic
2401 S. 31st St.
Temple, TX 76508
254-724-2554

UTAH

Intermountain Sleep
Disorders Ctr. of Murray
Cottonwood Hosp.
5770 South, 300 East
Murray, UT 84106
801-269-2015

Intermountain Sleep
Disorders Ctr.
LDS Hosp.
325 8th Ave.
Salt Lake City, UT 84143
801-321-3617

Sleep Disorders Ctr.
Univ. Health Sciences Ctr.
50 N. Med. Dr.
Salt Lake City, UT 84132
801-581-2016

VERMONT

No Accredited Member
Centers

VIRGINIA

Fairfax Sleep Disorders Ctr.
3289 Woodburn Rd., # 360
Annandale, VA 22003
703-876-9870

Virginia-Carolina Sleep
Disorders Ctr.
159 Executive Dr., # D
Danville, VA 24541
804-792-2209

Sleep Disorders Ctr.
Eastern Vir. Med. School
Sentara Norfolk Gen. Hosp.
600 Gresham Dr.
Norfolk, VA 23507
757-668-3322

Sleep Disorders Ctr.
Med. College of Virginia
P.O. Box 980710 - MCV
Richmond, VA 23298
804-828-1490

Sleep Disorders Ctr.
Carilion Roanoke
Comm. Hosp.
P.O. Box 12946
Roanoke, VA 24029
540-985-8526

Sleep Disorders Ctr.
Obici Hosp.
1900 N. Main St.
Suffolk, VA 23439
757-934-4450

Sleep Disorders Ctr.
Virginia Beach Gen. Hosp.
1060 First Colonial Rd.
Virginia Beach, VA 23454
757-481-8168

WASHINGTON

ARMC Sleep Apnea Lab*
Auburn Regional Med. Ctr.
Plaza One, 202 N. Division
Auburn, WA 98001
253-804-2809

St. Clare Sleep-Related
Breathing Disorders Clinic*
St. Clare Hosp.
11315 Bridgeport Way, S.W.
Lakewood, WA 98499
253-581-6951

Sleep Disorders Ctr. for
S.W. Washington
Providence St. Peter Hosp.
413 N. Lilly Rd.
Olympia, WA 98506
360-493-7436

Sleep Ctr. at Valley Med.
Ctr.
400 S. 43rd St.
Renton, WA 98055
425-656-5340

Columbia Sleep Lab*
780 Swift Blvd., # 130
Richland, WA 99352
509-943-6166

Richland Sleep
Disorders Ctr.
800 Swift Blvd., # 260
Richland, WA 99352
509-946-4632

Highline Sleep Disorder
Ctr.
Highline Comm. Hosp.
14212 Ambaum Blvd., S.W.
Seattle, WA 98166
206-325-7396

Providence Sleep
Disorders Ctr.
500 17th Ave., Dept. 4W
Seattle, WA 98122
206-320-2575

Seattle Sleep Disorders Ctr.
Swedish Med. Ctr./Ballard
P.O. Box 70707
Seattle, WA 98107
206-781-6359

Virginia Mason Med. Ctr.
Sleep Disorders Ctr.
Virginia Mason Hosp.
925 Seneca St.
Seattle, WA 98101
206-625-7180

Sleep Disorders Ctr.
Sacred Heart Doctors Bldg.
105 W. Eighth Ave., # 418
Spokane, WA 99204
509-455-4895

WEST VIRGINIA

Sleep Disorders Ctr.
Charleston Area Med. Ctr.
501 Morris St.
Charleston, WV 25325
304-348-7507

PM Sleep Medicine
3803 Emerson Ave.
Parkersburg, WV 26104
304-485-5041

WISCONSIN

Sleep Disorders Ctr.
Appleton Med. Ctr.
1818 N. Meade St.
Appleton, WI 54911
920-738-6460

Marshfield Clinic Sleep
Disorders Ctr.
2655 County Hwy. 1
Chippewa Falls, WI 54729
715-726-4136

Luther/Midelfort Sleep
Disorders Ctr.
Luther Hosp./Midelfort
Clinic
1221 Whipple St.
Eau Claire, WI 54702
715-838-3165

St. Vincent Hosp. Sleep
Disorders Ctr.
P.O. Box 13508
Green Bay, WI 54307
920-431-3041

Sleep Disorders Lab*
Bellin Hosp.
744 S. Webster Ave.
Green Bay, WI 54305
920-433-7441

Wisconsin Sleep
Disorders Ctr.
Gundersen Lutheran
1836 South Ave.
LaCrosse, WI 54601
608-782-7300

Comprehensive Sleep
Disorders Ctr. B6/579
Univ. of Wis. Hospitals
and Clinics
600 Highland Ave.
Madison, WI 53792
608-263-2387

Sleep Disorders Ctr.
St. Marys Hosp. Med. Ctr.
707 S. Mills St.
Madison, WI 53716
608-258-5266

Marshfield Sleep
Disorders Ctr.
Marshfield Clinic
1000 N. Oak Ave.
Marshfield, WI 54449
715-387-5397

Milwaukee Reg. Sleep
Disorders Ctr.
Columbia Hosp.
2025 East Newport Ave.
Milwaukee, WI 53211
414-961-4650

St. Luke's Sleep Disorders
Ctr.
St. Luke's Med. Ctr.
2801 W. Kinnickinnic River
Pkwy., # 445
Milwaukee, WI 53215
414-649-5288

WYOMING

No Accredited Member
Centers

APPENDIX TWO

Home Health Care Respiratory Therapists

The key to your success and health will be the nightly use of your CPAP. Your respiratory therapist will be a vital source of support and advice to make this significant change in your life as easy and comfortable for you as possible. The following list of highly recommended home care companies offering respiratory services was compiled by the author through interviews with American Sleep Disorder Association members.*

ALABAMA

American Home Patient
1996 Airport Blvd.
Alexander City, AL 35010
256-234-5036

American Home Patient
320 W. Bypass
Andalusia, AL 36420
334-222-6060

Anniston Health
930 Keith Ave.
Anniston, AL 36207
256-236-8126

Eagle Med. Eqpt.
915 S. Jefferson St.
Athens, AL 35611
256-771-0853

American Home Patient
102 Oxmoor Rd., # 126
Birmingham, AL 35209
205-942-9400

Apria Healthcare Inc.
100 Oxmoor Rd., # 104
Birmingham, AL 35209
205-942-4702

Birmingham Care
4100 Colonnade Pkwy.
Birmingham, AL 35243
205-969-1006

Hug Ctr.
104 Oxmoor Rd.
Birmingham, AL 35209
205-945-7055

PSA Home Healthcare
25 25th Ave., N.W.
Birmingham, AL 35215
205-853-2323

Specialized Med. Devices
1202 3rd Ave., S.E.
Birmingham, AL 35233
205-323-7400

Sand Mountain Med.
1068 Bethsadia Rd.
Boaz, AL 35957
256-593-0677

Southern Med.
110 3rd Ave., S.E.
Cullman, AL 35055
256-739-5915

Specialized Med. Devices
2418 Danville Rd., S.W.
Decatur, AL 35603
256-353-2881

American Home Patient
1236 W. Main St.
Dothan, AL 36301
334-793-2978

Baumanns
1023 Oates St.
Dothan, AL 36301
334-794-3174

American Home Patient
309 Fayette Square
Shopping Ctr.
Fayette, AL 35555
501-932-5974

*In order to keep our information current for future editions, we welcome submissions from additonal home health care respiratory therapists for consideration.

American Home Patient
1113 N. Mckenzie St.
Foley, AL 36535
334-943-5821

Fuller Med. Co
524 Broad St.
Gadsden, AL 35901
256-547-4991

NMC Homecare
2106 Rainbow Dr.
Gadsden, AL 35901
256-549-1911

Physicians Home Health
214 S. 5th St.
Gadsen, AL 35901
256-546-8820

Rainbow Med.
1601 W. Meighan Blvd.
Gadsden, AL 35901
256-546-6319

American Home Patient
714 Madison St., S.E.
Huntsville, AL 35801
256-533-1628

Apria Healthcare Inc.
5000 Whitesburg Dr., S
Huntsville, AL 35802
256-880-2875

Southern Med.
2313 Whitesburg Dr., S
Huntsville, AL 35801
256-533-4454

Specialized Med. Devices
805 Madison St., S.E., # 1B
Huntsville, AL 35801
256-536-7676

American Home Patient
7 McGregor Ave., S.
Mobile, AL 36608
334-380-5280

Apria Healthcare Inc.
4970 Rangeline Rd.
Mobile, AL 36619
334-665-5200

Lincare
602 Bel Air Blvd., # 11
Mobile, AL 36606
334-473-5122

American Home Patient
2801 Vaughn Plaza Rd., # T `
Montgomery, AL 36116
334-277-9933

Lincare
131 Market Pl., # A
Montgomery, AL 36117
334-260-0124

American Home Patient
1515 2nd Ave.
Opelika, AL 36801
334-749-4904

Anniston Health
30 Plaza Ln.
Oxford, AL 36203
205-831-2215

Caretenders
283 Cahaba Vall. Pkwy., N.
Pelham, AL 35124
205-978-5200

Eagle Med.
129 Rana Dr., # 8B
Pinckard, AL 36371
334-983-4804

American Home Patient
107 N. Broadway Ave.
Sylacauga, AL 35150
256-245-1119

American Home Patient
Victorian Village
Sylacauga, AL 35150
256-245-2226

American Home Patient
1005 Hwy. 231
Troy, AL 36081
334-566-0712

American Home Patient
610 Parkview Ctr.
Tuscaloosa, AL 35401
205-349-1204

Caretenders
2020 Canyon Rd.
Vestavia Hills, AL 35216
205-822-4411

ALASKA

Apria Healthcare Inc.
2000 W. Intl Airport Rd.
Anchorage, AK 99502
907-248-8484

Northwest Med.
2401 E. 42nd Ave., # 204
Anchorage, AK 99508
907-563-0073

Apria Healthcare Inc.
3512 International St.
Fairbanks, AK 99701
907-458-8912

Apria Healthcare Inc.
44539 Sterling Hwy.
Soldotna, AK 99669
907-260-3505

ARIZONA

Lincare
559 W. 4th St.
Benson, AZ 85602
520-586-7911

Apria Healthcare Inc.
2400 Hwy. 95
Bullhead City, AZ 86442
520-763-7787

Apria Healthcare Inc.
1355 E. Florence Blvd.
Casa Grande, AZ 85222
520-836-2300

American Home Patient
1417 E. U.S. Hwy. 89A
Cottonwood, AZ 86326
520-639-0980

Apria Healthcare Inc.
295 S. Willard St., # 101
Cottonwood, AZ 86326
520-634-7528

Apria Healthcare Inc.
1500 E. Cedar Ave.
Flagstaff, AZ 86004
520-773-9493

American Home Patient
1100 N. Broad St.
Globe, AZ 85501
520-425-5795

Apria Healthcare Inc.
1300 Russel Rd.
Globe, AZ 85501
520-425-3113

American Home Patient
2370 Northern Ave.
Kingman, AZ 86401
520-692-7747

Lincare
1134 E. University Dr.
Mesa, AZ 85203
602-610-2822

Apria Healthcare Inc.
806 S. Ponderosa St.
Payson, AZ 85541
520-474-6293

American Home Patient
4040 E. Raymond St.
Phoenix, AZ 85040
602-784-2217

Apria Healthcare Inc.
2202 E. University Dr.
Phoenix, AZ 85034
602-438-0000

Lincare
2850 S. 36th St.
Phoenix, AZ 85034
602-437-3372

NMC Homecare
3844 E. University Dr., # 4
Phoenix, AZ 85034
602-437-4480

Osco Home Health
439 S. 55th St.
Phoenix, AZ 85043
602-274-4452

American Home Patient
1030 Sandretto Dr.
Prescott, AZ 86301
520-778-7772

Apria Healthcare Inc.
1841 E. State Route 69
Prescott, AZ 86301
520-445-0477

Lincare
1365 Iron Springs Rd., # A5
Prescott, AZ 86301
520-708-0202

NMC Homecare
172 E. Merritt St., # A
Prescott, AZ 86301
520-771-0167

Advent Home Health
7302 E. Helm Dr.
Scottsdale, AZ 85260
602-998-9600

Apria Healthcare Inc.
4481 S. White Mountain
Rd.
Show Low, AZ 85901
520-537-7330

Apria Healthcare Inc.
999 E. Fry Blvd., # 101
Sierra Vista, AZ 85635
520-452-1382

American Home Patient
3939 S. Park Ave.
Tucson, AZ 85714
520-746-3330

Apria Healthcare Inc.
2850 E. Valencia Rd.
Tucson, AZ 85706
520-295-5980

Lincare
1020 E. Palmdale St., # 110
Tucson, AZ 85714
520-795-8161

NMC Homecare
4455 S. Park Ave.
Tucson, AZ 85714
520-889-0143

American Home Patient
2375 S. 4th Ave.
Yuma, AZ 85364
520-343-1256

Apria Healthcare Inc.
2185 E. Palo Verde St.
Yuma, AZ 85365
520-782-6509

ARKANSAS

Southern Med.
910 Clay St.
Arkadelphia, AR 71923
870-246-5303

American Home Patient
1699 Harrison St.
Batesville, AR 72501
870-793-6567

Southern Med.
103 S. Freeman St.
Dermott, AR 71638
870-538-3272

Lincare
2850 N. College Ave.
Fayetteville, AR 72703
501-442-8401

PSA Home Healthcare
125 E. Township St., # 4
Fayetteville, AR 72703
501-443-0625

Lincare
4720 Rogers Ave.
Fort Smith, AR 72903
501-484-0505

Lincare
515 N. Main St.
Harrison, AR 72601
870-365-7468

American Home Patient
1820 Higdon Ferry Rd., # E
Hot Springs, AR 71913
501-321-2200

Southern Med.
1018 Airport Rd.
Hot Springs, AR 71913
501-767-0002

American Home Patient
824 Cobb St.
Jonesboro, AR 72401
870-972-1580

American Home Patient
3005 Middlefield Dr.
Jonesboro, AR 72401
870-935-8222

American Home Patient
15 Shackleford Dr., # F
Little Rock, AR 72211
501-221-3479

Lincare
6701 W. 12th St., # 5
Little Rock, AR 72204
501-664-2525

PSA Home Healthcare
1601 Westpark Dr., # 1
Little Rock, AR 72204
501-663-3600

American Home Patient
318 S. 10th St.
Paragould, AR 72450
870-239-2101

Lincare
3139 W. 28th Ave.
Pine Bluff, AR 71603
870-862-8900

Lincare
3005 Hawkins Dr.
Searcy, AR 72143
501-268-3588

Duracare Med.
1209 S. Thompson St.
Springdale, AR 72764
501-872-1488

CALIFORNIA

American Home Health
245 E. Main St.
Alhambra, CA 91801
626-457-9825

NMC Homecare
13620 Lincoln Way
Auburn, CA 95603
530-823-2984

Apria Healthcare Inc.
1314 34th St.
Bakersfield, CA 93301
805-324-4887

Lincare
2000 Truxtun Ave.
Bakersfield, CA 93301
805-335-0400

NMC Homecare
5329 Office Ctr. Ct.
Bakersfield, CA 93309
805-635-3052

Apria Healthcare Inc.
977 Armory Rd.
Barstow, CA 92311
760-252-4555

Apria Healthcare Inc.
1369 Rocking Dr., W.
Bishop, CA 93514
760-872-1866

Lincare
201 N. Hollywood Way
Burbank, CA 91505
818-503-0497

Lincare
614 S. Glenwood Pl.
Burbank, CA 91506
818-407-0202

Homedco Inc.
393 E. Hamilton Ave.
Campbell, CA 95008
408-295-6285

Lincare
Capitola, CA 95010
408-724-5010

Apria Healthcare Inc.
909 E. 236th St.
Carson, CA 90745
310-212-7168

NMC Homecare
20765 Superior St..
Chatsworth, CA 91311
818-700-1266

Apria Healthcare Inc.
3028 Esplanade
Chico, CA 95973
530-891-5226

Lincare
2505 Zanella Way, # B
Chico, CA 95928
530-895-8414

Lincare
2961 Hwy. 32
Chico, CA 95973
530-895-0151

Apria Healthcare Inc.
14860 Olympic Dr.
Clearlake, CA 95422
707-994-1236

Apria Healthcare Inc.
4095 Pike Ln.
Concord, CA 94520
510-827-8800

Home Med
5046 Commercial Dr.
Concord, CA 94520
510-680-0638

Apria Healthcare Inc.
3560 Hyland Ave.
Costa Mesa, CA 92626
714-957-2000

Apria Healthcare Inc.
630 G St.
Crescent City, CA 95531
707-464-4242

Apria Healthcare Inc.
6200 Enterprise Dr.
Diamond Spgs, CA 95619
530-642-4240

Apria Healthcare Inc.
401 W. Main St.
El Centro, CA 92243
760-353-6465

Apria Healthcare Inc.
1735 2nd St.
Eureka, CA 95501
707-444-8022

Apria Healthcare Inc.
910 W. Texas St.
Fairfield, CA 94533
707-428-3300

Lincare
1861 Walters Ct., # A
Fairfield, CA 94533
707-422-7757

Lincare
3 Juniper Ln., # 2
Fall River Mills, CA 96028
530-336-6761

Apria Healthcare Inc.
301 E. Redwood Ave.
Fort Bragg, CA 95437
707-961-1770

Apria Healthcare Inc.
4747 N. Bendel Ave., # 104
Fresno, CA 93722
559-277-0263

Apria Healthcare Inc.
4762 W. Jennifer Ave.
Fresno, CA 93722
559-276-0733

Lincare
6700 N. 1st St., # 116
Fresno, CA 93710
559-435-6379

NMC Homecare
2212 N. Winery Ave., # 101
Fresno, CA 93703
559-252-0200

Advent Home Health
Box 1128
Glendora, CA 91740
626-852-1985

Medmart
555 S. Vermont
Glendora, CA 91741
626-963-0620

Apria Healthcare Inc.
6464 Hollister Ave.
Goleta, CA 93117
805-965-6050

Apria Healthcare Inc.
2547 Barrington Ct.
Hayward, CA 94545
510-786-1860

NMC Homecare
3521 Investment Blvd.
Hayward, CA 94545
510-732-5487

Apria Healthcare Inc.
43301 Division St., # 312
Lancaster, CA 93535
805-949-3447

NMC Homecare
43423 Division St.
Lancaster, CA 93535
805-948-0660

Sierra Home Care
2451 Foothill Blvd.
La Verne, CA 91750
909-596-3330

Apria Healthcare Inc.
697 N. H St.
Lompoc, CA 93436
805-735-3402

Home Respiratory Care
2370 Westwood Blvd., # D
Los Angeles, CA 90064
310-441-4640

Advent Home Health
718 Univ. Ave.
Los Gatos, CA 95030
408-399-4800

Apria Healthcare Inc.
2260 Cooper Ave., # B
Merced, CA 95348
209-384-7100

CPAP Co.
500 E. Calaveras
Milpitas, CA 95035
408-935-8170

Apria Healthcare Inc.
4400 Sisk Rd.
Modesto, CA 95356
209-545-8540

Lincare Inc.
1705 Coffee Rd.
Modesto, CA 95355
209-522-4985

Apria Healthcare Inc.
1 Lower Ragsdale Bldg.
Monterey, CA 93940
831-757-5444

Sierra Home Care
12125 Day St.
Moreno Valley, CA 92557
909-320-1420

Lincare
Morgan Hill, CA 95037
408-779-9221

Apria Healthcare Inc.
1220 Trancas St.
Napa, CA 94558
707-257-3775

Special Respiratory
18327 Napa St.
Northridge, CA 91325
818-717-8807

Apria Healthcare Inc.
12950 E. Alondra Blvd.
Norwalk, CA 90650
562-921-1850

Bay Area Health
385 Bel Marin Keys
Novato, CA 94949
415-883-7980

Tru-Care
61 Galli Dr.
Novato, CA 94949
415-884-2384

Gemmel Med.
137 N. Euclid
Ontario, CA 91762
909-984-9112

Inland Valley Resp.
350 S. Milliken
Ontario, CA 91761
909-390-9956

NMC Homecare
2143 E. D St.
Ontario, CA 91764
909-984-9711

Apria Healthcare Inc.
2150 Trabajo Dr.
Oxnard, CA 93030
805-983-0926

Palisades Homecare
1515 Palisades Dr., # M
Pacific Palisades, CA 90272
310-459-9888

Lincare
44710 San Pablo Ave.
Palm Desert, CA 92260
760-346-7488

Apria Healthcare Inc.
1243 N. Gene Autry Trl.
Palm Springs, CA 92262
760-778-5366

Lincare
383 N. Indian Canyon Dr.
Palm Springs, CA 92262
760-922-8122

Lincare
1111 Riverside Ave.
Paso Robles, CA 93446
805-239-4045

Apria Healthcare Inc.
19698 State Hwy. 88
Pine Grove, CA 95665
209-296-4206

Lincare
1166 Broadway
Placerville, CA 95667
530-642-5454

Apria Healthcare Inc.
590 W. Putnam Ave.
Porterville, CA 93257
209-781-0991

Lincare
344 S. Main St.
Red Bluff, CA 96080
530-529-4141

Apria Healthcare Inc.
2706 S. Market St., # A
Redding, CA 96001
530-243-8772

Lincare
1620 E. Cypress Ave., # 12
Redding, CA 96002
530-223-2080

American Home Health
25814 Business Ctr. Dr.
Redlands, CA 92374
909-799-8488

Apria Healthcare Inc.
9960 Indiana Ave., # 9
Riverside, CA 92503
909-785-5400

Apria Healthcare Inc.
1880 Iowa Ave.
Riverside, CA 92507
909-686-6222

NMC Homecare
1830 Sierra Gardens Dr.
Roseville, CA 95661
916-783-9886

Apria Healthcare Inc.
4244 S. Market Ct., # A
Sacramento, CA 95834
916-927-5400

John Davis Co.
3412 Auburn Blvd.
Sacramento, CA 95821
916-484-1591

Lincare
1431 N. Market Blvd., # 1
Sacramento, CA 95834
916-928-9350

Lincare
1000 S. Main St., # 313
Salinas, CA 93901
831-758-1934

Lincare
365 Victor St., # I
Salinas, CA 93907
831-758-4612

Lincare
720 Carnegie Dr., # 260
San Bernardino, CA 92408
909-889-6767; 814-6673

NMC Homecare
1832 Commercenter Cir.
San Bernardino, CA 92408
909-890-1577

American Home Health
9520 Padgett St.
San Diego, CA 92126
619-536-5525

Apria Healthcare Inc.
9115 Activity Rd., # 100
San Diego, CA 92126
619-653-6800

Coram Healthcare
8804 Balboa Ave.
San Diego, CA 92123
619-576-6969

Lincare
13230 Evening Creek Dr., S
San Diego, CA 92128
619-486-8555

Apria Healthcare Inc.
555 1st St.
San Fernando, CA 91340
818-999-0088

Apria Healthcare Inc.
480 Carlton Ct.
San Francisco, CA 94103
415-588-9744

Apria Healthcare Inc.
2040 Corporate Ct.
San Jose, CA 95131
408-866-2311

Lincare
1370 Tully Rd., # 504
San Jose, CA 95122
408-286-1026

Advanced Respiratory Care
2953 Teagarden St.
San Leandro, CA 94577
510-895-4403

Apria Healthcare Inc.
2995 McMillan Ave., # 196
San Luis Obispo, CA 93401
805-546-0208

Apria Healthcare Inc.
356 Santa Rosa St.
San Luis Obispo, CA 93405
805-541-0111

Lincare
2925 McMillan Ave., # 124
San Luis Obispo, CA 93401
805-434-2947

Lincare
3070 Kerner Blvd., # D
San Rafael, CA 94901
415-457-0407

American Home Health
1950 E. 17th St.
Santa Ana, CA 92705
714-550-0800

Apria Healthcare Inc.
115 S. La Cumbre Ln.
Santa Barbara, CA 93105
805-687-9222

Apria Healthcare Inc.
1334 Brommer St., # B3
Santa Cruz, CA 95062
831-465-0281

Lincare
427 W. Betteravia Rd., # B
Santa Maria, CA 93455
805-928-5731

Apria Healthcare Inc.
3636 N. Laughlin Rd.
Santa Rosa, CA 95403
707-543-0921

Apria Healthcare Inc.
480 Carlton Ct.
South San Francisco, CA
94080
650-588-9744

Homedco
512 S. Airport Blvd.
South San Francisco, CA
94080
650-467-5990

Homedco
480 Carlton Ct.
South San Francisco, CA
94080
650-872-7930

Lincare
874 Dubuque Ave.
South San Francisco, CA
94080
650-952-6969

Lincare
920 N. Yosemite St.
Stockton, CA 95203
209-957-1339

Bay Area Health
7906 Foothill Blvd.
Sunland, CA 91040
310-829-1778

Bay Area Health
275 N. Mathilda
Sunnyvale, CA 94086
650-941-9600

Lincare
2807 Oregon Ct.
Torrance, CA 90503
310-328-7322

Bay Area Health
Box 65
Tujunga, CA 91043
818-951-6701

Apria Healthcare Inc.
2521 Michelle Dr.
Tustin, CA 92780
949-978-2330

Apria Healthcare Inc.
221 E. Gobbi St.
Ukiah, CA 95482
707-468-9242

Apria Healthcare Inc.
30116 Eigenbrodt Way
Union City, CA 94587
510-483-3500

Apria Healthcare Inc.
14464 Atstar Dr., # 101
Victorville, CA 92392
760-241-4488

Apria Healthcare Inc.
1526 E. Mineral King Ave.
Visalia, CA 93292
559-732-6040

Apguard
6325 Desoto Ave.
Woodland Hills, CA 91367
818-713-1874

Lincare
1525 Lucas Rd., # B
Yreka, CA 96097
530-841-0503

Apria Healthcare Inc.
990 Klamath Ln., # 11
Yuba City, CA 95993
530-673-5513

Lincare
951 Live Oak Blvd.
Yuba City, CA 95991
530-649-2814

Lincare
990 Klamath Ln.
Yuba City, CA 95993
530-755-0200

COLORADO

Apria Healthcare Inc.
445 Poncha Ave.
Alamosa, CO 81101
719-589-2551

Apria Healthcare Inc.
6325 Corporate Dr.
Colorado Springs, CO
80919
719-594-9090

Lincare
921 E. Fillmore St.
Colorado Springs, CO
80907
719-630-0202

NMC Homecare
4179 Sinton Rd.
Colorado Springs, CO
80907
719-593-2950

PSA Home Healthcare
1110 Elkton Dr., # B
Colorado Springs, CO
80907
719-536-9790

American Home Patient
1850 E. Main St.
Cortez, CO 81321
970-565-3204

American Home Health
1873 S. Bellaire St., # 800
Denver, CO 80222
303-782-5111

Lincare
7000 E. 47th Ave., # 900
Denver, CO 80216
303-377-5800

American Home Patient
1802 Main Ave.
Durango, CO 81301
970-259-5106

Apria Healthcare Inc.
3206 Main Ave.
Durango, CO 81301
970-259-7575

Lincare
4400 S. Federal Blvd.
Englewood, CO 80110
303-730-3058

Lincare
3500 S. Corona St.
Englewood, CO 80110
303-377-0202

Lincare
8200 S. Akron St.
Englewood, CO 80112
303-799-8441

NMC Homecare
7032 S. Revere Pkwy.
Englewood, CO 80112
303-790-0271

Lincare
555 Prospect Ave.
Estes Park, CO 80517
970-586-8447

Apria Healthcare Inc.
1337 Riverside Ave.
Fort Collins, CO 80524
970-484-8211

Lincare
1001 S. Lemay Ave.
Fort Collins, CO 80524
970-482-8114

Lincare
322 E. Railroad Ave., # B
Fort Morgan, CO 80701
970-542-1516

Apria Healthcare Inc.
210 Ctr. Dr
Glenwood Spgs, CO 81601
970-945-5648

Lincare
51241 Hwy. 6
Glenwood Spgs, CO 81601
970-945-1450

PSA Home Healthcare
2001 Blake Ave.
Glenwood Spgs, CO 81601
970-945-2888

Apria Healthcare Inc.
666 Patterson Rd.
Grand Junction, CO 81506
970-245-1604

PSA Home Healthcare
1048 Independent Ave.
Grand Junction, CO 81505
970-241-7744

Apria Healthcare Inc.
1675 18th Ave.
Greeley, CO 80631
970-353-5355

Lincare
802 16th Ave.
Greeley, CO 80631
970-356-1506

Lincare
210 Santa Fe Ave.
La Junta, CO 81050
719-384-2554

Lincare
220 S. Main St.
Lamar, CO 81052
719-336-4940

Apria Healthcare Inc.
300 E. Mineral Ave., # 2
Littleton, CO 80122
303-428-5055

Apria Healthcare Inc.
385 S. Pierce Ave., # A
Louisville, CO 80027
303-604-2249

Lincare
686 S. Taylor Ave., # 103
Louisville, CO 80027
303-604-1222

Apria Healthcare Inc.
1714 Topaz Dr.
Loveland, CO 80537
970-663-0500

PSA Home Healthcare
Monte Vista, CO 81144
719-852-3477

Apria Healthcare Inc.
1205 S. Townsend Ave.
Montrose, CO 81401
970-249-7733

American Home Patient
68 Bastille Dr., # 4
Pagosa Springs, CO 81147
970-731-5480

Apria Healthcare Inc.
607 N. Santa Fe Ave.
Pueblo, CO 81003
719-545-1690

Lincare
301 N. Santa Fe Ave.
Pueblo, CO 81003
719-542-4654

Roth Med.
729 W. Fortino Blvd.
Pueblo, CO 81008
719-544-1414

PSA Home Healthcare
2128 Railroad Ave.
Rifle, CO 81650
970-625-0111

Lincare
134 W. Main St.
Trinidad, CO 81082
719-846-7648

PSA Home Healthcare
Vail, CO 81657
970-476-9742

Apria Healthcare Inc.
341 Main St.
Wray, CO 80758
970-332-3310

CONNECTICUT

Lincare
61 Commerce Dr.
Brookfield, CT 06804
203-775-6551

Lincare
72 Grays Bridge Rd., # E
Brookfield, CT 06804
203-748-1022

PSA Home Healthcare
1172 Post Rd.
Fairfield, CT 06430
203-256-4346

Lincare
77 Kreiger Ln., # 804
Glastonbury, CT 06033
860-657-3033

Apria Healthcare Inc.
5 Hamden Park Dr.
Hamden, CT 06517
203-288-7938

Lincare
464 Pratt St. Ext.
Meriden, CT 06450
203-634-1264

American Home Patient
182 S. Main St.
New Britain, CT 06051
860-223-8325

Apria Healthcare Inc.
91 Holmes Rd.
Newington, CT 06111
860-666-6199

Lincare
70 Howard St.
New London, CT 06320
860-442-8252

Apria Healthcare Inc.
20 Murphy Rd.
North Franklin, CT 06254
860-886-2486

Lincare
22 Corporate Dr.
North Haven, CT 06473
203-239-3113

Lincare
26 Pearl St.
Norwalk, CT 06850
203-849-0400

NMC Homecare
900 N. Northrop Rd., # F
Wallingford, CT 06492
203-294-9744

Apria Healthcare Inc.
141 South St.
West Hartford, CT 06110
860-493-6200

Lincare
612 Quaker Ln., S., # B
West Hartford, CT 06110
860-236-4586

DELAWARE

American Home Patient
321 Independence Blvd.
Dover, DE 19904
302-537-0524

American Home Patient
311 Ruthar Dr.
Newark, DE 19711
302-454-3390

Apria Healthcare Inc.
225 Lake Dr.
Newark, DE 19702
302-737-7979

American Home Patient
16 Trolley Sq., # A
Wilmington, DE 19806
302-654-8181

FLORIDA

Lincare
224 W. Central Pkwy.
Altamonte Spgs, FL 32714
407-846-4144

Lincare
43 S. Desoto Ave.
Arcadia, FL 34266
941-993-9787

Lincare
910 Oakfield Dr.
Brandon, FL 33511
813-651-4425

NMC Homecare
739 E. Brandon Blvd.
Brandon, FL 33511
813-654-4389

Lincare
10141 Cortez Blvd.
Brooksville, FL 34613
352-596-5400

Apria Healthcare Inc.
1126 S.E. 12th Ct.
Cape Coral, FL 33990
941-574-5525

Lincare
4910 Creekside Dr.
Clearwater, FL 33760
727-573-5911

Lincare
4700 140th Ave., N.
Clearwater, FL 33762
727-538-0908

Lincare
19361 U.S. Hwy. 19, N.
Clearwater, FL 33764
727-530-7800

Lincare
19337 U.S. Hwy. 19 N.
Clearwater, FL 33764
727-530-7700

American Home Patient
3055 Crawfordville Hwy.
Crawfordville, FL 32327
850-926-7497

American Home Patient
1420 Mason Ave.
Daytona Beach, FL 32117
904-274-4000

Lincare
270 S.W. 12th Ave.
Deerfield Beach, FL 33442
954-481-6686

NMC Homecare
1350 E. Newport Ctr. Dr.
Deerfield Beach, FL 33442
954-427-7200

Lincare
1812 Main St.
Dunedin, FL 34698
727-733-2927

Caretenders
1500 N.W. 62nd St.
Fort Lauderdale, FL 33309
954-267-9696

PSA Home Healthcare
6460 N.W. 5th Way
Fort Lauderdale, FL 33309
954-772-1630

American Home Patient
1853 Commercial Dr.
Fort Myers, FL 33901
941-936-2717

American Home Patient
501 Goodlette Rd., # C104
Fort Myers, FL 33901
941-261-2717

Lincare
13891 Jetport Loop, # 6
Fort Myers, FL 33913
941-768-2422

American Home Patient
3715 N.W. 97th Blvd.
Gainesville, FL 32606
352-376-3848

Lincare
237 S.W. 7th Ter.
Gainesville, FL 32601
352-335-7390

Lincare
1607 N. Nova Rd., # A
Holly Hill, FL 32117
904-673-6868

Apria Healthcare Inc.
3351 Executive Way
Hollywood, FL 33025
954-450-7270

Apria Healthcare Inc.
16550 Scheer Blvd., # 3
Hudson, FL 34667
727-336-1882

Apria Healthcare Inc.
3802 E. Gulf To Lake Hwy.
Inverness, FL 34453
352-637-2211

Lincare
1110 Sterling Rd.
Inverness, FL 34450
352-726-6400

American Home Patient
8182 Baymeadows Way W.
Jacksonville, FL 32256
904-296-2472

Apria Healthcare Inc.
9143 Phillips Hwy.
Jacksonville, FL 32256
904-363-3200

Lincare
6128 Kennerly Rd.
Jacksonville, FL 32216
904-739-2385

NMC Homecare
2700 University Blvd., W.
Jacksonville, FL 32217
904-733-4600

Lincare
2316 Lakeland Hills Blvd.
Lakeland, FL 33805
941-688-4888

Lincare
1135 Lakeland Hills Blvd.
Lakeland, FL 33805
941-688-7717

Lincare
7217 Bryan Dairy Rd.
Largo, FL 33777
727-545-3717

American Home Patient
2245 Citrus Blvd.
Leesburg, FL 34748
352-867-0087

Lincare
1635 Timocuan Way
Longwood, FL 32750
407-339-6116

All-Care
804 E. Hibiscus
Melbourne, FL 32901
407-727-1400

Apria Healthcare Inc.
274 N. Wickham Rd.
Melbourne, FL 32935
407-255-3534

Browning's Healthcare
141 E. Hibiscus Blvd.
Melbourne, FL 32901
407-725-6320

Lincare
1520 S. Babcock St.
Melbourne, FL 32901
407-254-0082

Rotech Oxygen
380 N. Wickham Rd.
Melbourne, FL 32935
407-752-1100

NMC Homecare
9360 Sunset Dr.
Miami, FL 33173
305-477-7777

Lincare
935 3rd Ave., N.
Naples, FL 34102
941-261-7290

Lincare Inc
2902 N.E. 23rd St.
Ocala, FL 34470
352-629-8880

Lincare
117 S.W. Park St.
Okeechobee, FL 34972
941-763-7337

Apria Healthcare Inc.
3443 Parkway Ctr. Ct.
Orlando, FL 32808
407-297-0100

Healthcare Eqpt.
2405 McRae Ave.
Orlando, FL 32803
407-898-6004

Signature Home Health
715 State Rd. 434, # J
Oviedo, FL 32765
407-850-9065

American Home Patient
316 U.S. Hwy. 19 S.
Palatka, FL 32177
904-325-9880

American Home Patient
617 N. Hwy. 231
Panama City, FL 32405
850-763-6861

Lincare
2250 Jenks Ave.
Panama City, FL 32405
850-769-4700

American Home Patient
2720 N. Palafox St.
Pensacola, FL 32501
850-435-4778

Apria Healthcare Inc.
3636 N. L St., # D
Pensacola, FL 32505
850-433-7434

Lincare
5700 N. Davis Hwy., # 6
Pensacola, FL 32503
850-478-9141

Lincare
1701 S. Alexander St., # 112
Plant City, FL 33567
813-752-5683

Gold Coast Respiratory
4100 N. Powerline Rd.
Pompano Beach, FL 33073
954-776-6862

Lincare
2450 Tamiami Trl., # A
Port Charlotte, FL 33952
941-625-2530

Lincare
8403 Redmac St.
Port Richey, FL 34668
813-843-0164

American Home Patient
1430 S.W. St. Lucie West
Blvd.
Port St. Lucie, FL 34986
561-871-2753

American Home Patient
1335 S. U.S. 1
Rockledge, FL 32955
407-632-3515

American Home Patient
1937 State Rd. 3
St. Augustine, FL 32084
904-471-2011

NMC Homecare
10901 Roosevelt Blvd. N.
St. Petersburg, FL 33716
727-576-7070

Apria Healthcare Inc.
327 Interstate Blvd.
Sarasota, FL 34240
941-377-5458

Lincare
999 Cattlemen Rd.
Sarasota, FL 34232
941-378-1553

Apria Healthcare Inc.
6406 U.S. Hwy. 27 S.
Sebring, FL 33870
941-382-4540

Lincare
4163 U.S. Hwy. 27 S.
Sebring, FL 33870
941-382-9292

Apria Healthcare Inc.
7882 S.W. Ellipse Way
Stuart, FL 34997
561-283-8700

Lincare
4020 Sun City Ctr. Blvd.
Sun City, FL 33573
813-633-0722

American Home Patient
1307 N. Monroe St.
Tallahassee, FL 32303
850-222-1723

Lincare
1962 Village Green Way
Tallahassee, FL 32308
850-385-6594

American Home Patient
6313 Benjamin Rd., # 106
Tampa, FL 33634
813-885-9578

Apria Healthcare Inc.
5414 Beaumont Ctr. Blvd.
Tampa, FL 33634
813-885-5568

Homedco
9834 Currie Davis Dr.
Tampa, FL 33619
813-626-1437

Lincare
10770 N. 46th St., # C300
Tampa, FL 33617
813-971-3449

Lincare
1109 Lake Harris Dr.
Tavares, FL 32778
352-742-1955

American Home Patient
357 Cypress Dr.
Tequesta, FL 33469
561-743-1266

Lincare
130 S. U.S. Hwy. 1
Vero Beach, FL 32962
561-567-0822

Apria Healthcare Inc.
2200 N. Florida Mango Rd.
West Palm Beach, FL 33409
561-471-3030

Lincare
2100 45th St., # B1
West Palm Beach, FL 33407
561-842-2333

NMC Homecare
901 Northpoint Pkwy.
West Palm Beach, FL 33407
561-615-8860

Apria Healthcare Inc.
3629 Havendale Blvd.,
N.W.
Winter Haven, FL 33881
941-324-2838

Lincare
1164 Solana Ave.
Winter Park, FL 32789
407-645-3161

Lincare
6948 Gall Blvd.
Zephyrhills, FL 33541
813-780-7155

GEORGIA

American Home Patient
2316 N. Slappey Blvd.
Albany, GA 31701
912-432-2027

Apria Healthcare Inc.
4555 Mansell Rd., # 220
Alpharetta, GA 30022
770-433-1800

American Home Patient
1530 E. Forsyth St., # D
Americus, GA 31709
912-924-1987

Apria Healthcare Inc.
8601 Dunwoody Pl.
Atlanta, GA 30350
404-587-0638

PSA Home Healthcare
1021 15th St.
Augusta, GA 30901
706-724-7771

American Home Patient
3610 Altama Ave.
Brunswick, GA 31520
912-264-5333

PSA Home Healthcare
108 Barnes Ave.
Carrollton, GA 30117
770-834-6003

PSA Home Healthcare
3228 University Ave., # 108
Columbus, GA 31907
706-561-5251

Apria Healthcare Inc.
958 McEver Rd.
Gainesville, GA 30504
770-536-4770

PSA Home Healthcare
1062 Thompson Ct.
Gainesville, GA 30501
770-531-1014

CS Med.
135 Macon W.
Macon, GA 31210
912-475-0013

American Home Patient
821 Livingston Ct. S.E., # D
Marietta, GA 30067
770-419-5994

American Home Patient
476 Flowing Wells Rd.
Martinez, GA 30907
706-868-0695

Lincare
1319 S. Main St
Moultrie, GA 31768
912-891-2803

American Home Patient
509 S. Davis St.
Nashville, GA 31639
912-686-3407

Apria Healthcare Inc.
70 Bullsboro Dr.
Newnan, GA 30263
770-251-6550

Hi-Tech Homecare
5980 Unity Dr.
Norcross, GA 30071
770-449-6785

Homedco
5555 Oakbrook Pkwy.
Norcross, GA 30093
770-587-0615

Lincare
3230 Peachtree Corners
Norcross, GA 30092
770-662-5105

Oxy-Plus
5300 Oakbrook Pkwy.
Norcross, GA 30093
770-806-8000

PSA Home Healthcare
6145 Northbelt Pkwy.
Norcross, GA 30071
770-263-6373

American Home Patient
306 Cloud Springs Rd.
Rossville, GA 30741
706-861-0903

American Home Patient
5007 Paulsen St.
Savannah, GA 31405
912-353-7400

PSA Home Healthcare
206 Currahee St.
Toccoa, GA 30577
706-282-1421

American Home Patient
2803 N. Ashley St.
Valdosta, GA 31602
912-244-2467

American Home Patient
1905 Tebeau St.
Waycross, GA 31501
912-285-8355

HAWAII

Apria Healthcare Inc.
Hilo, HI 96720
808-969-1211

Respiratory Homecare
805 Pahukaina
Honolulu, HI 96813
808-592-1400

Apria Healthcare Inc.
251 Lalo St., # A1
Kahului, HI 96732
808-871-4267

Pacific Island Med.
328 Ilimano St.
Kailua, HI 96734
808-254-1300

Apria Healthcare Inc.
74 Alapa St., # 7
Kailua Kona, HI 96740
808-329-8911

Kohala Home Health
64 Mamalahoa Hwy.
Kamuela, HI 96743
808-885-9126

Kohala Home Health
Akoni Pule Hwy., #6
Kapaau, HI 96755
808-889-5406

Oxy Med Hawaii
712 California Ave.
Wahiawa, HI 96786
808-622-6944

IDAHO

Lincare
5557 Kendall St.
Boise, ID 83706
208-463-8227

Norco Med.
400 Main St.
Boise, ID 83702
208-344-7933

Lincare
296 W. Sunset Ave., # 18
Coeur d'Alene, ID 83815
208-765-3422

Apria Healthcare Inc.
1626 17th
Lewiston, ID 83501
208-743-1267

Mercy Homecare
1311 12th Ave.
Nampa, ID 83686
208-465-6511

Whitmore Med.
3135 Kimberly Rd.
Twin Falls, ID 83301
208-733-6270

ILLINOIS

American Home Patient
5630 W. 120th St.
Alsip, IL 60803
708-239-4200

American Home Patient
3860 N. Ventura Dr.
Arlington Hts., IL 60004
847-590-1212

Apria Healthcare Inc.
5807 N. Belt W.
Belleville, IL 62226
618-277-5251

Apria Healthcare Inc.
1103 Martin Luther King Dr.
Bloomington, IL 61701
309-827-0011

Dependicare
1815 Gardner Rd.
Broadview, IL 60153
708-345-7400

Apria Healthcare Inc.
8120 S. Madison St.
Burr Ridge, IL 60521
630-920-0044

Apria Healthcare Inc.
234 W. Cerro Gordo St.
Decatur, IL 62522
217-428-2180

Apria Healthcare Inc.
3453 Rupp Pkwy.
Decatur, IL 62526
217-876-8940

Apria Healthcare Inc.
565 Lamont Rd.
Elmhurst, IL 60126
630-941-6400

Homedco
655 W. Grand Ave.
Elmhurst, IL 60126
630-941-6400

American Home Health
500 Park Blvd., # 190C
Itasca, IL 60143
630-285-0555

Apria Healthcare Inc.
1132 Veterans Dr.
Jacksonville, IL 62650
217-243-5807

Apria Healthcare Inc.
2302 Oak Leaf St.
Joliet, IL 60436
815-741-0494

Apria Healthcare Inc.
10910 N. 2nd St.
Machesney Park, IL 61115
815-624-8671

Apria Healthcare Inc.
1909 W. Coolidge Ave., # B
Marion, IL 62959
765-997-6469

American Home Patient
8226 N. University St.
Peoria, IL 61615
309-691-7200

Apria Healthcare Inc.
7708 N. Harker Dr.
Peoria, IL 61615
309-691-1012

Apria Healthcare Inc.
926 Broadway
Quincy, IL 62301
217-228-1595

Rockford Health
4223 E. State St.
Rockford, IL 61108
815-971-3550

Ventilatory Care
3402 N. Rockton Ave.
Rockford, IL 61103
815-877-4357

Apria Healthcare Inc.
5320 Mainsail Dr.
Roscoe, IL 61073
815-633-4400

American Home Patient
2908 Old Rochester Rd.
Springfield, IL 62703
217-753-1525

Apria Healthcare Inc.
2837 Singer Ave.
Springfield, IL 62703
217-789-0461

Apria Healthcare Inc.
1410 N. Bloomington St.
Streator, IL 61364
815-672-5683

Apria Healthcare Inc.
1502 N. Cunningham Ave.
Urbana, IL 61802
217-367-8383

Apria Healthcare Inc.
49 E. Edwardsville Rd.
Wood River, IL 62095
618-254-0701

INDIANA

Apria Healthcare Inc.
3802 Industrial Blvd., # 3
Bloomington, IN 47403
812-333-9901

Lincare
420 W. 2nd St.
Bloomington, IN 47403
812-339-5579

Caretenders
590 Missouri Ave., # 202
Clarksville, IN 47129
812-285-9266

Apria Healthcare Inc.
2101 Maxwell Ave.
Evansville, IN 47711
812-471-0202

Caretenders
1222 Professional Blvd.
Evansville, IN 47714
812-471-4100

Apria Healthcare Inc.
7515 Westfield Dr.
Fort Wayne, IN 46825
219-489-7722

Lincare
1200 Airport Office Park N.
Fort Wayne, IN 46825
219-489-0481

American Home Health
8849 Shelby St.
Indianapolis, IN 46227
317-859-2900

Apria Healthcare Inc.
1400 N. Ritter Ave., # 140
Indianapolis, IN 46219
317-355-1355

Apria Healthcare Inc.
7353 Company Dr.
Indianapolis, IN 46237
317-865-4200

Indiana Respiratory
5335 N. Tacoma Ave., #20
Indianapolis, IN 46220
317-251-1144

Lincare
3530 S. Keystone Ave.
Indianapolis, IN 46227
317-786-7909

Lincare
4245 S. High School Rd.
Indianapolis, IN 46241
317-856-8841

NMC Homecare
7998 Georgetown Rd.
Indianapolis, IN 46268
317-297-9616

Lincare
304 E. Court Ave.
Jeffersonville, IN 47130
812-285-0177

Apria Healthcare Inc.
711 S. Reed Rd.
Kokomo, IN 46901
765-457-6613

Lincare
902 S. Reed Rd.
Kokomo, IN 46901
765-452-4627

Apria Healthcare Inc.
1160 S. Creasy Ln.
Lafayette, IN 47905
765-448-9995

Lincare
2504 Greenbush St.
Lafayette, IN 47904
765-449-4198

Apria Healthcare Inc.
1581 E. 90th Pl.
Merrillville, IN 46410
219-879-2882

Lincare
1575 E. 89th Ave., # C
Merrillville, IN 46410
219-755-0130

Apria Healthcare Inc.
810 Park Pl.
Mishawaka, IN 46545
219-277-7850

Apria Healthcare Inc.
4401 W. Williamsburg Blvd.
Muncie, IN 47304
765-286-8017

Lincare
5752 W. Kilgore Ave.
Muncie, IN 47304
765-747-0477

Lincare
2019 Chester Blvd.
Richmond, IN 47374
765-962-3424

Apria Healthcare Inc.
1714 N. 5th St.
Terre Haute, IN 47804
812-232-0267

Lincare
556 E. Springhill Dr.
Terre Haute, IN 47802
812-232-0651

Apria Health Care
1000 S. Main St.
Tipton, IN 46072
765-675-8577

Lincare
701 S. 13th St.
Vincennes, IN 47591
812-886-0367

IOWA

NMC Homecare
108 5th Ave., S.W.
Altoona, IA 50009
515-967-7633

Apria Healthcare Inc.
213 Duff Ave.
Ames, IA 50010
515-233-0044

Apria Healthcare Inc.
609 N. Court St.
Carroll, IA 51401
712-792-6022

NMC Homecare
220 1st Ave.
Coralville, IA 52241
319-351-0558

Apria Healthcare Inc.
701 W. Townline St.
Creston, IA 50801
515-782-6892

Apria Healthcare Inc.
351 W. 76th St.
Davenport, IA 52806
319-388-9530

NMC Homecare
1006 Central Ave.
Fort Dodge, IA 50501
515-576-8027

Apria Healthcare Inc.
220 Lafayette St.
Iowa City, IA 52240
319-338-7373

Hamilton Med.
817 S. Gilbert St.
Iowa City, IA 52240
319-354-6149

Apria Healthcare Inc.
1515 Blairs Ferry Rd.
Marion, IA 52302
319-377-3199

American Home Patient
616 S. Monroe Ave.
Mason City, IA 50401
515-423-7500

Apria Healthcare Inc.
1140 N. Jefferson St., # 216
Ottumwa, IA 52501
515-682-8088

Apria Healthcare Inc.
111 Washington Ave.
Red Oak, IA 51566
712-623-5466

Apria Healthcare Inc.
2400 Pierce St.
Sioux City, IA 51104
712-255-1555

NMC Homecare
2200 W. 19th St.
Sioux City, IA 51103
712-252-1678

Apria Healthcare Inc.
125 Flindt Dr.
Storm Lake, IA 50588
712-732-7710

Apria Healthcare Inc.
11224 Aurora Ave.
Urbandale, IA 50322
515-270-0536

Apria Healthcare Inc.
2530 Falls Ave.
Waterloo, IA 50701
319-232-1525

KANSAS

Apria Healthcare Inc.
1255 S. Country Club Dr.
Colby, KS 67701
785-462-8661

Apria Healthcare Inc.
408 W. Frontview St.
Dodge City, KS 67801
316-225-9008

Apria Healthcare Inc.
306 E. 23rd St.
Fort Scott, KS 66701
316-223-6015

Homedco
Oldfort Blvd., # 2
Fort Scott, KS 66701
316-365-7223

Apria Healthcare Inc.
2009 Vine St.
Hays, KS 67601
785-628-6080

Lincare
840 S. Washington St.
Junction City, KS 66441
785-238-4554

Lincare
104 Greystone Ave.
Kansas City, KS 66103
913-371-3377

Apria Healthcare Inc.
9500 Widmer Rd.
Lenexa, KS 66215
913-492-2212

NMC Homecare
9301 W. 53rd St.
Merriam, KS 66203
913-384-2100

NMC Homecare
5800 Foxridge Dr., # 200
Mission, KS 66202
913-599-5300

Lincare
2411 Main St.
Parsons, KS 67357
316-421-2774

American Home Patient
2401 N. Broadway St.
Pittsburg, KS 66762
316-232-3452

Apria Healthcare Inc.
1109 W. Crawford St.
Salina, KS 67401
785-823-9235

American Home Health
6701 W. 64th St., # 109
Shawnee Mission, KS 66202
913-384-4323

Apria Healthcare Inc.
1505 S.W. 6th Ave.
Topeka, KS 66606
785-234-3681

Knoll Patient Supply
1112 S.W. 6th Ave.
Topeka, KS 66606
785-232-5972

Signature Home Care
631 N.W. Tyler Ct.
Topeka, KS 66608
785-235-1500

American Home Health
731 N. McLean Blvd., # 120
Wichita, KS 67203
316-942-3400

Apria Healthcare Inc.
7803 E. Osie St., # 101
Wichita, KS 67207
316-689-4500

Lincare
535 N. Woodlawn St.
Wichita, KS 67208
316-684-4689

KENTUCKY

Caretenders
208 W. John Fitch Ave.
Bardstown, KY 40004
502-349-1728

A-1 Healthcare
411 Fairfield Ave.
Bellevue, KY 41073
606-655-9940

American Home Patient
830 Fairview Ave.
Bowling Green, KY 42101
502-781-6050

Apria Healthcare Inc.
1051 Bryant Way
Bowling Green, KY 42103
502-781-2787

Caretenders
Hwy. 1051 Bypass Rd.
Brandenburg, KY 40108
502-422-5090

American Home Patient
1005 18th St.
Corbin, KY 40701
606-523-5100

Caretenders
2865 Chancellor Dr.
Covington, KY 41017
606-578-0022

Rothert
2020 Madison Ave.
Covington, KY 41014
606-431-5900

American Home Patient
975 Hustonville Rd., # 11
Danville, KY 40422
606-238-7777

Caretenders
424 S. 4th St.
Danville, KY 40422
606-236-1717

American Home Patient
227 Main St.
Eddyville, KY 42038
502-388-4870

American Home Patient
1515 Ring Rd., # 4
Elizabethtown, KY 42701
502-737-0403

Caretenders
1002 Woodland Dr.
Elizabethtown, KY 42701
502-765-4422

American Home Patient
7505 Sussex Dr.
Florence, KY 41042
606-283-1115

Caretenders
410 Kings Daughters Dr.
Frankfort, KY 40601
502-226-3537

Caretenders
129 2nd St.
Henderson, KY 42420
502-826-3860

American Home Patient
Rockhouse Creek Rd.
Hyden, KY 41749
606-672-3638

American Home Patient
726 Kentucky Hwy. 15 N.
Jackson, KY 41339
606-666-8869

Caretenders
259 W. Walnut St.
Lebanon, KY 40033
502-692-0550

Caretenders
105 N. Main St.
Leitchfield, KY 42754
502-259-2994

American Home Patient
1510 Newtown Pike
Lexington, KY 40511
606-254-7102

Bluegrass Oxygen
366 Waller Ave., # 104
Lexington, KY 40504
606-277-2583

Caretenders
2432 Regency Rd.
Lexington, KY 40503
606-278-7700

Lovejoy Med.
171 Prosperous Pl.
Lexington, KY 40509
606-263-2587

American Home Patient
3307 Gilmore Indus. Blvd.
Louisville, KY 40213
502-968-1751

Apria Healthcare Inc.
1805 Taylor Ave.
Louisville, KY 40213
502-454-3550

Caretenders
100 Mallard Creek Rd.
Louisville, KY 40207
502-425-2273

Health Care Partners
10500 Bluegrass Pkwy.
Louisville, KY 40299
502-499-9099

Holdaway's
11400 Bluegrass Pkwy.
Louisville, KY 40299
502-266-0092

American Home Patient
301 Sturgis Rd.
Marion, KY 42064
502-965-9859

American Home Patient
Meally, KY 41234
606-789-2172

Caretenders
994 N. Main St.
Nicholasville, KY 40356
606-885-5055

Caretenders
5000 Back Square Dr.
Owensboro, KY 42301
502-685-3876

American Home Patient
116 Lone Oak Rd.
Paducah, KY 42001
502-443-8727

Caretenders
2017 Main St.
Paris, KY 40361
606-987-0517

Cooley Med. Eqpt.
536 S. Mayo Trail
Pikeville, KY 41501
606-432-0055

American Home Patient
110 Kentucky Ave.
Pineville, KY 40977
606-337-6680

CDS Home Care
5459 Kentucky Route 321
Prestonburg, KY 41653
606-886-8155

Resp-A-Care
956 Commercial Dr.
Richmond, KY 40475
606-623-2202

American Home Patient
90 Southport Dr.
Somerset, KY 42501
606-679-2000

Caretenders
142 Chenoweth Ln.
St. Matthews, KY 40207
502-896-1444

LOUISIANA

Apria Healthcare Inc.
11871 Dunlay Ave.
Baton Rouge, LA 70809
225-751-8668

Apria Healthcare Inc.
6730 Exchequer Dr.
Baton Rouge, LA 70809
225-751-8668

Lincare
7434 Town South Ave.
Baton Rouge, LA 70808
225-755-0888

American Home Patient
213 Superior Ave.
Bogalusa, LA 70427
504-732-0004

Southern Med.
2207 California Dr.
Bossier City, LA 71111
318-742-9853

Southern Med.
105 Illinois St.
Delhi, LA 71232
318-878-2402

American Home Patient
42014 Veterans Ave.
Hammond, LA 70403
504-542-4343

Apria Healthcare Inc.
4740 W. Congress St.
Lafayette, LA 70506
318-981-9993

Lincare
505 Loire Ave.
Lafayette, LA 70507
318-896-3388

Apria Healthcare Inc.
1830 Ryan St., # E
Lake Charles, LA 70601
318-433-8103

Apria Healthcare Inc.
2113 Justice St.
Monroe, LA 71201
318-322-9911

Lincare
1203 Royal Ave.
Monroe, LA 71201
318-325-6467

Apria Healthcare Inc.
1510 Kuebel St.
New Orleans, LA 70123
504-734-0563

Lincare
5701 Crawford St., # B
New Orleans, LA 70123
504-733-1702

Apria Healthcare Inc.
5203 Interstate Dr.
Shreveport, LA 71109
318-631-6701

Apria Healthcare Inc.
2535 Bert Kouns Ind. Loop
Shreveport, LA 71118
318-445-0850

Lincare
1303 Line Ave.
Shreveport, LA 71101
318-226-0555

American Home Patient
101 Commercial Square
Slidell, LA 70461
504-649-1045

Lincare
1503 Gause Blvd.
Slidell, LA 70458
504-643-5472

MAINE

Apria Healthcare Inc.
100 Dowd Rd.
Bangor, ME 04401
207-942-5579

Apria Healthcare Inc.
22 Birdseye Ave., # C
Caribou, ME 04736
207-496-2120

Lincare
4 Fundy Rd. Rear
Falmouth, ME 04105
207-781-5551

NMC Homecare
160 Larrabee Rd., # C
Westbrook, ME 04092
207-856-2266

Apria Healthcare Inc.
14 Yarmouth Jct.
Yarmouth, ME 04096
207-846-8543

Homedco
44 N. Elm St.
Yarmouth, ME 04096
207-846-8500

MARYLAND

Lincare
1589 Sulphur Spring Rd.
Baltimore, MD 21227
410-247-7676

Apria Healthcare Inc.
12400 Kiln Ct.
Beltsville, MD 20705
301-419-2061

NMC Homecare
6935 Oakland Mills Rd.
Columbia, MD 21045
410-381-0770

American Home Patient
505 N. Centre St.
Cumberland, MD 21502
301-722-6300

American Home Patient
1 Wormans Mill Ct.
Frederick, MD 21701
301-695-5000

Apria Healthcare Inc.
919 Sweeney Dr.
Hagerstown, MD 21740
301-791-5500

Accu-Care
11 Gwynns Mill Ct.
Owings Mills, MD 21117
410-581-7900

Mid Atlantic Healthcare
11407 Cron Hill Dr.
Owings Mills, MD 21117
410-356-1414

PSA Home Healthcare
1700 Reisterstown Rd.
Pikesville, MD 21208
410-486-3800

American Home Patient
207 Milford St.
Salisbury, MD 21804
410-742-3711

Apria Healthcare Inc.
307 Winfield Ave.
Salisbury, MD 21801
410-742-8383

MASSACHUSETTS

Apria Healthcare Inc.
208 Southbridge St.
Auburn, MA 01501
508-832-9666

Lincare
143 Oxford St., N.
Auburn, MA 01501
508-832-9013

Caretenders
187 Billerica Rd.
Chelmsford, MA 01824
978-250-1212

Lincare
69 Main St.
Cherry Valley, MA 01611
508-892-9367

Lincare
155 Webster St.
Hanover, MA 02339
781-871-7799

Lincare
69 S. Main St.
Leicester, MA 01524
508-754-3342

Apria Healthcare Inc.
575 University Ave.
Norwood, MA 02062
781-255-7600

Apria Healthcare Inc.
170 Carando Dr.
Springfield, MA 01104
413-736-4529

Apria Healthcare Inc.
1658 GAR Hwy., # 3
Swansea, MA 02777
508-677-1700

Lincare
8 Filko Ave., # 5
Swansea, MA 02777
508-379-0050

Lincare
25 Capital Dr.
West Springfield, MA 01089
413-734-2562

Apria Healthcare Inc.
260 Fordham Rd.
Wilmington, MA 01887
978-657-8443

Lincare
17 Everberg Rd., # D
Woburn, MA 01801
781-938-9311

MICHIGAN

Apria Healthcare Inc.
1099 Highland Dr., # C
Ann Arbor, MI 48108
734-973-8144

Apria Healthcare Inc.
820 Capital Ave., S.W.
Battle Creek, MI 49015
616-965-7287

Apria Healthcare Inc.
2280 South M139
Benton Harbor, MI 49022
616-925-3440

Apria Healthcare Inc.
411 W. 5th St.
Clare, MI 48617
517-773-1268

Apria Healthcare Inc.
1323 Ludington St.
Escanaba, MI 49829
906-789-1303

Airway Oxygen
2935 Madison Ave., S.E.
Grand Rapids, MI 49548
616-247-3900

Apria Healthcare Inc.
1840 Wealthy St., S.E.
Grand Rapids, MI 49506
616-774-7553

Apria Healthcare Inc.
4513 Broadmoor Ave., S.E.
Grand Rapids, MI 49512
616-698-9119

Apria Healthcare Inc.
704 Sharon Ave.
Houghton, MI 49931
906-482-3041

Apria Healthcare Inc.
9851 U.S. Hwy. 31
Interlochen, MI 49643
616-938-2702

Apria Healthcare Inc.
116 S. Merritt Ave.
Iron Mountain, MI 49801
906-779-1892

Apria Healthcare Inc.
606 E. Michigan Ave.
Jackson, MI 49201
517-787-6989

Apria Healthcare Inc.
921 Portage St.
Kalamazoo, MI 49001
616-342-0022

White & White
5121 E. M.L. Ave.
Kalamazoo, MI 49001
616-345-2011

Airway Oxygen
739 Brookside Dr.
Lansing, MI 48917
517-321-4747

Apria Healthcare Inc.
4310 S. Creyts Rd.
Lansing, MI 48917
517-322-0617

Apria Healthcare Inc.
4728 W. U.S. Hwy. 10
Ludington, MI 49431
616-845-1273

Apria Healthcare Inc.
1414 W. Fair Ave.
Marquette, MI 49855
906-228-2230

Apria Healthcare Inc.
2011 10th St..
Menominee, MI 49858
906-863-4481

American Home Health
135 W. Auburn Rd.
Rochester, MI 48307
248-844-9122

Apria Healthcare Inc.
600 E. Morley Dr.
Saginaw, MI 48601
517-752-0141

Classic Med.
22919 E. Industrial Dr.
St. Clair Shores, MI 48080
810-774-1450

Apria Healthcare Inc.
103 W. Sanilac Rd.
Sandusky, MI 48471
810-648-4404

Apria Health Care
6005 Miller Rd.
Swartz Creek, MI 48473
810-635-0440

Apria Healthcare Inc.
1199 S. U.S. Hwy. 23
Tawas City, MI 48763
517-362-8695

Apria Healthcare Inc.
1755 Maplelawn Dr.
Troy, MI 48084
248-643-4140

American Home Health
14200 E. 11 Mile Rd., # B
Warren, MI 48089
810-445-9600

Mitchell Home Med.
4811 Carpenter Rd.
Ypsilanti, MI 48197
734-570-0203

MINNESOTA

Apria Healthcare Inc.
701 N. 6th Ave., E.
Duluth, MN 55805
218-723-7121

Apria Healthcare Inc.
131 Cheshire Ln.
Minnetonka, MN 55305
612-404-1500

Apria Healthcare Inc.
1500 Opportunity Rd.,
N.W.
Rochester, MN 55901
507-285-0065

Apria Healthcare Inc.
451 W. Saint Germain St.
St. Cloud, MN 56301
320-251-4611

MISSISSIPPI

Apria Healthcare Inc.
2198 Pass Rd.
Biloxi, MS 39531
228-385-2200

Apria Healthcare Inc.
101 Hwy. 51 N.
Brookhaven, MS 39601
601-833-1500

Apria Healthcare Inc.
112 Hwy. 9 N.
Eupora, MS 39744
601-258-2985

Apria Healthcare Inc.
200 N. 40th Ave.
Hattiesburg, MS 39401
601-264-3111

Apria Healthcare Inc.
2715 N. State St.
Jackson, MS 39216
601-362-0523

Lincare
811 Foley St., # G
Jackson, MS 39202
601-354-1144

Apria Healthcare Inc.
1312 22nd Ave.
Meridian, MS 39301
601-485-4551

American Home Patient
1040 Cliff Gookin Blvd.
Tupelo, MS 38801
601-842-1100

MISSOURI

American Home Patient
309 N. Walnut St.
Cameron, MO 64429
816-632-2183

American Home Patient
63 Doctors Park
Cape Girardeau, MO 63703
573-339-1980

Apria Healthcare Inc.
1405 N. Mount Auburn Rd.
Cape Girardeau, MO 63701
573-334-4207

Apria Healthcare Inc.
107 S. Washington St.
Clinton, MO 64735
660-885-8129

American Home Patient
3208 Lemone Indus. Blvd.
Columbia, MO 65201
573-442-8877

Apria Healthcare Inc.
502 Earth City Plaza, # 204
Earth City, MO 63045
314-522-2849

American Home Patient
1302 S. Aurora St.
Eldon, MO 65026
573-392-1400

Apria Healthcare Inc.
2694 U.S. Hwy. 67
Farmington, MO 63640
573-756-6761

American Home Patient
622 Collins Dr.
Festus, MO 63028
314-937-7607

American Home Patient
2307 Broadway
Hannibal, MO 63401
573-221-7603

NMC Homecare
201 S. Grand Ave.
Houston, MO 65483
417-967-3818

American Home Patient
111 S. Main St.
Ironton, MO 63650
573-546-3993

American Home Patient
1515 W. 10th St., # E
Joplin, MO 64801
417-623-1700

Apria Healthcare Inc.
1122 Illinois Ave., # 104
Joplin, MO 64801
417-782-6212

Lincare
2617 Cunningham Ave.
Joplin, MO 64804
417-782-5959

NMC Homecare
1602 E. 20th St.
Joplin, MO 64804
417-782-1939

American Home Patient
7028 Universal Ave.
Kansas City, MO 64120
816-333-0033

Apria Healthcare Inc.
1001 N.W. Chipman Rd.
Lees Summit, MO 64081
816-554-9630

Lincare
5 Worthington Access Dr.
Maryland Hts., MO 63043
314-878-0202

Lincare
929 Fee Fee Rd.
Maryland Hts., MO 63043
314-205-0077

American Home Patient
1007 W. Monroe St.
Mexico, MO 65265
573-581-9808

NMC Homecare
614 W. Jackson St.
Mexico, MO 65265
573-581-1721

American Home Patient
100 W. 17th St., # D
Mountain Grove, MO 65711
417-926-4000

NMC Homecare
1901 Belt Way Dr.
Overland, MO 63114
314-428-7171

American Home Patient
6 Parkway Ctr.
Potosi, MO 63664
573-438-2000

Apria Healthcare Inc.
4416 S. 40th St.
St. Joseph, MO 64503
816-233-2449

NMC Homecare
4908 Frederick Ave.
St. Joseph, MO 64506
816-233-6477

American Home Patient
7435 Watson Rd., # 76
St. Louis, MO 63119
314-961-4770

Apria Healthcare Inc.
8248 Lackland Rd.
St. Louis, MO 63114
314-968-1616

Apria Healthcare Inc.
2727 Hereford St.
St. Louis, MO 63139
314-773-0773

American Home Patient
3045 E. Chestnut Expy.
Springfield, MO 65802
417-869-6708

American Home Patient
1447 S. Enterprise Ave.
Springfield, MO 65804
417-883-2125

Apria Healthcare Inc.
1601 W. Sunshine St., # C
Springfield, MO 65807
417-866-1727

NMC Homecare
2102 W. Vista St.
Springfield, MO 65807
417-881-6994

American Home Patient
610 E. Young Ave.
Warrensburg, MO 64093
660-747-7135

Homedco
7790 Watson Rd.
Webster Groves, MO 63119
314-968-8224

MONTANA

Lincare
547 S. 20th St. W., # 3
Billings, MT 59102
406-652-0771

NEBRASKA

Homedco
1201 S. 9th St.
Beatrice, NE 68310
402-228-3972

Apria Healthcare Inc.
300 King St.
Chadron, NE 69337
308-432-3256

NMC Homecare
143 E. Roberts St.
Grand Island, NE 68803
308-381-7030

Apria Healthcare Inc.
715 N. Saint Joseph Ave.
Hastings, NE 68901
402-463-2320

Apria Healthcare Inc.
3700 2nd Ave.
Kearney, NE 68847
308-236-6619

Apria Healthcare Inc.
1631 Cushman Dr.
Lincoln, NE 68512
402-434-2950

Bryan Home Med.
1600 S. 48th St.
Lincoln, NE 68506
402-483-3888

Capital Med.
145 S. 66th St.
Lincoln, NE 68510
402-484-7373

Apria Healthcare Inc.
711 E. 11th St.
McCook, NE 69001
308-345-2477

Apria Healthcare Inc.
214 E. 5th St.
North Platte, NE 69101
308-534-7733

NMC Homecare
509 E. 7th St.
North Platte, NE 69101
308-532-2366

Apria Healthcare Inc.
5505 F St.
Omaha, NE 68117
402-731-8700

Koley's
8646 F St.
Omaha, NE 68127
402-331-5472

NMC Homecare
8603 G St.
Omaha, NE 68127
402-339-7572

NMC Homecare
320 E. Douglas St.
O'Neill, NE 68763
402-336-1619

Apria Healthcare Inc.
3912 Avenue B
Scottsbluff, NE 69361
308-632-3559

NEVADA

Lincare
151 E. Park St.
Carson City, NV 89706
775-882-0333

Apria Healthcare Inc.
1250 Lamoille Hwy.
Elko, NV 89801
775-738-3808

Apria Healthcare Inc.
1435 Industrial Way
Gardnerville, NV 89410
702-782-3011

Apria Healthcare Inc.
3955 W. Mesa Vista Ave.
Las Vegas, NV 89118
702-736-4466

Lincare
5701 W. Charleston Blvd.
Las Vegas, NV 89102
702-878-9200

NMC Homecare
3321 Sunrise Ave.
Las Vegas, NV 89101
702-438-2273

Sierra Home Care
1755 E. Plumb Ln.
Reno, NV 89502
775-348-7573

Apria Healthcare Inc.
1395 Greg St., # 113
Sparks, NV 89431
775-352-7742

Lincare
1380 Greg St.
Sparks, NV 89431
775-359-6262

NEW HAMPSHIRE

Lincare
6 Chenell Dr.
Concord, NH 3301
603-224-3507

Keene Med.
240 Meriden Rd.
Lebanon, NH 3766
603-448-5225

Apria Healthcare Inc.
915 Holt Ave.
Manchester, NH 3109
603-625-2133

Lincare
951 Islington St.
Portsmouth, NH 3801
603-749-5563

NEW JERSEY

NMC Homecare
5 Terri Ln., # 14
Burlington, NJ 08016
609-239-7588

Lincare
2428 Route 38
Cherry Hill, NJ 08002
609-482-2500

American Home Patient
30 Concordia Shopping Ctr.
Cranbury, NJ 08512
609-655-3111

Take Good Care
1800 Rt. 27
Edison, NJ 08817
732-819-9611

Apria Healthcare Inc.
2628 Fire Rd., # 301
Egg Harbor Twp., NJ 08234
609-641-8000

Apria Healthcare Inc.
170 Oberlin Ave., N.
Lakewood, NJ 08701
732-905-1400

Apria Healthcare Inc.
1 Frassetto Way, # F
Lincoln Park, NJ 07035
973-305-0099

Apria Healthcare Inc.
118 Burrs Rd., # C
Mt Holly, NJ 08060
609-265-2190

Lincare
1340 Campus Pkwy.
Neptune, NJ 07753
732-919-7400

Lincare
286 U.S. Hwy. 46
Parsippany, NJ 07054
973-808-9515

NMC Homecare
45 U.S. Hwy. 46, # 602
Pine Brook, NJ 07058
973-227-5623

Apria Healthcare Inc.
1500 Wildwood Blvd.
Rio Grande, NJ 08242
609-465-9003

NEW MEXICO

American Home Patient
1001 10th St.
Alamogordo, NM 88310
505-434-3778

Lincare Inc
804 10th St.
Alamogordo, NM 88310
505-437-6155

Apria Healthcare Inc.
4401 McLeod Rd., N.E.
Albuquerque, NM 87109
505-881-9111

**Highland American Home
Patient**
300 Central Ave., S.E.
Albuquerque, NM 87102
505-243-5664

Lincare
101 Sin Nombre Ct., N.E.
Albuquerque, NM 87113
505-344-6760

NMC Homecare
5571 Midway Park, N.E.
Albuquerque, NM 87109
505-345-7904

Lincare
830 N. Main St.
Belen, NM 87002
505-864-2202

Lincare
1117 W. Pierce St.
Carlsbad, NM 88220
505-885-4116

American Home Patient
1010 W. 21st St.
Clovis, NM 88101
505-762-2964

Apria Healthcare Inc.
1202 W. 21st St.
Clovis, NM 88101
505-763-0202

Lincare
2201 Columbus Rd.
Deming, NM 88030
505-546-4647

American Home Patient
906 San Juan Blvd.
Farmington, NM 87401
505-326-9193

Apria Healthcare Inc.
1020 N. Butler Ave.
Farmington, NM 87401
505-325-7575

Lincare
713 E. Roosevelt Ave.
Grants, NM 87020
505-876-6186

American Home Patient
1034 E. Bender Blvd.
Hobbs, NM 88240
505-392-8217

Apria Healthcare Inc.
2827 N. Dal Paso St., # 101
Hobbs, NM 88240
505-392-0202

American Home Patient
1132 S. Solano Dr.
Las Cruces, NM 88001
505-523-8572

Apria Healthcare Inc.
210 E. Idaho Ave., # B
Las Cruces, NM 88005
505-525-2494

Lincare
2285 E. Lohman Ave.
Las Cruces, NM 88001
505-525-2423

American Home Patient
901 W. 2nd St.
Roswell, NM 88201
505-622-5612

Apria Healthcare Inc.
604 E. College Blvd.
Roswell, NM 88201
505-622-4747

Lincare
205 W. 6th St.
Roswell, NM 88201
505-622-1112

Apria Healthcare Inc.
1570 Pacheco St., # D-6
Santa Fe, NM 87505
505-982-2901

Lincare
712 W. San Mateo Rd.
Santa Fe, NM 87505
505-992-8286

NMC Homecare
1225 Parkway Dr., # A
Santa Fe, NM 87505
505-474-6469

Lincare
320 California St.
Socorro, NM 87801
505-835-0859

NMC Homecare
212 Paseo Del Canon, # A
Taos, NM 87571
505-758-3075

NEW YORK

American Home Patient
501 New Karner Rd.
Albany, NY 12205
518-452-7017

Apria Healthcare Inc.
12 Petra Ln.
Albany, NY 12205
518-452-0445

Lincare
2 Access Rd.
Albany, NY 12205
518-869-4120

American Home Patient
Depot Rd.
Auburn, NY 13021
315-253-0543

American Home Patient
1159 Abbott Rd.
Buffalo, NY 14220
716-827-3700

American Home Patient
6816 Ellicott Dr.
East Syracuse, NY 13057
315-463-7299

Apria Healthcare Inc.
6327 E. Molloy Rd.
East Syracuse, NY 13057
315-463-5217

Apria Healthcare Inc.
452 E. Water St.
Elmira, NY 14901
607-732-5225

Lincare
1225 W. Water St.
Elmira, NY 14905
607-732-1126

Apria Healthcare Inc.
3 Westchester Plaza
Elmsford, NY 10523
914-592-1410

Apria Healthcare Inc.
3116 Watson Blvd.
Endwell, NY 13760
607-754-3511

Apria Healthcare Inc.
110 Bi County Blvd., # 122
Farmingdale, NY 11735
516-293-1440

Apria Healthcare Inc.
10905 14th Ave.
Flushing, NY 11356
718-358-8854

Lincare
5917 S. Park Ave.
Hamburg, NY 14075
716-648-3100

Lincare
5 Skyline Dr.
Hawthorne, NY 10532
914-592-8700

Lincare
328 N. Meadow St.
Ithaca, NY 14850
607-277-4027

Lincare
796 Fairmount Ave.
Jamestown, NY 14701
716-484-1292

Apria Healthcare Inc.
625 Sawkill Rd.
Kingston, NY 12401
914-336-3333

Lincare
4 Airport Park Blvd.
Latham, NY 12110
518-782-7700

Lincare
292 N. Plank Rd.
Newburgh, NY 12550
914-562-5800

NMC Homecare
587 Main St.
New York Mills, NY 13417
315-736-3303

Lincare
824 Proctor Ave.
Ogdensburg, NY 13669
315-393-6480

NMC Homecare
900 Champlain St.
Ogdensburg, NY 13669
315-393-4767

American Home Patient
5626 State Route 7, # 4
Oneonta, NY 13820
607-432-7757

Lincare
446 Main St.
Oneonta, NY 13820
607-432-8280

American Home Patient
140 Village Square
Painted Post, NY 14870
607-962-3115

NMC Homecare
675 Route 3
Plattsburgh, NY 12901
518-561-1420

Lincare
154 Pike St.
Port Jervis, NY 12771
914-856-6955

Apria Healthcare Inc.
75 Market St.
Potsdam, NY 13676
315-265-1161

Apria Health Care
1250 Scottsville Rd.
Rochester, NY 14624
716-436-4910

Lincare
939 Jefferson Rd.
Rochester, NY 14623
716-424-5640

American Home Patient
833 W. Genesee St.
Skaneateles, NY 13152
315-685-8000

Lincare
476 E. Brighton Ave.
Syracuse, NY 13210
315-472-0461

Lincare
1307 Champlin Ave.
Utica, NY 13502
315-793-8945

Lincare
732 Vestal Pkwy. E.
Vestal, NY 13850
607-757-0584

American Home Patient
1511 Washington St.
Watertown, NY 13601
315-788-3488

Lincare
22622 Murrock Circle
Watertown, NY 13601
315-785-3681

NMC Homecare
2500 Shames Dr.
Westbury, NY 11590
516-876-2121

Apria Healthcare Inc.
1975 Wehrle Dr.
Williamsville, NY 14221
716-631-1192

Apria Healthcare Inc.
1 Odell Plaza
Yonkers, NY 10701
914-375-0323

NORTH CAROLINA

Apria Healthcare Inc.
44 Buck Shoals Rd., # B1
Arden, NC 28704
704-684-9981

American Home Patient
1209 N. Fayetteville St.
Asheboro, NC 27203
336-625-1010

American Home Patient
1636 Hendersonville Rd.
Asheville, NC 28803
828-277-7514

Lincare
312 Ridgefield Ct.
Asheville, NC 28806
828-665-8389

American Home Patient
111 Mitchell Ave.
Bakersville, NC 28705
704-688-9110

Lincare
378 North Carolina Hwy.
105 Bypass, # 3
Boone, NC 28607
828-297-1786

American Home Patient
3411 Saint Vardell Ln., # B
Charlotte, NC 28217
704-529-1924

Apria Healthcare Inc.
1901 Crossbeam Dr., # D
Charlotte, NC 28217
704-329-0523

Caretenders of Charlotte
3700 Latrobe Dr.
Charlotte, NC 28211
704-366-1422

Lincare
2848 S. I-85 Service Rd.
Charlotte, NC 28208
704-391-9111

NMC Homecare
5025 W. W.T. Harris Blvd.
Charlotte, NC 28269
704-597-4100

Apria Healthcare Inc.
5594 Cumberland Rd.
Fayetteville, NC 28306
910-426-4000

Lincare
230 Sloan Rd.
Franklin, NC 28734
704-349-3151

Apria Healthcare Inc.
4249 Piedmont Pkwy.
Greensboro, NC 27410
336-767-9556

Apria Healthcare Inc.
702 W.H. Smith Blvd., # A
Greenville, NC 27834
252-757-1727

Lincare
669 S. Memorial Dr.
Greenville, NC 27834
252-758-6532

Apria Healthcare Inc.
415 Western Blvd., # B
Jacksonville, NC 28546
910-455-9322

Lincare
203 N. Main St.
Jefferson, NC 28640
336-246-4944

PSA Home Healthcare
2024 Connelly Spgs Rd.
S.W.
Lenoir, NC 28645
704-726-1306

American Home Patient
2700 Gateway Centre Blvd.
Morrisville, NC 27560
919-481-1550

Apria Healthcare Inc.
2600 Perimeter Park Dr.
Morrisville, NC 27560
919-380-1180

Lincare
991 Aviation Pkwy., # 400
Morrisville, NC 27560
919-481-3690

American Home Patient
1618 Millers Gap Hwy.
Newland, NC 28657
704-898-9070

Lincare
1913 W. Park Dr.
No. Wilkesboro, NC 28659
336-838-7515

Apria Healthcare Inc.
165 Page Rd.
Pinehurst, NC 28374
910-295-3175

American Home Health
3420 Tarheel Dr.
Raleigh, NC 27609
919-876-4336

American Home Patient
408 Summit Dr.
Sanford, NC 27330
919-774-2385

American Home Patient
442 E. Main St.
Sylva, NC 28779
704-586-8781

American Home Patient
114 E. Wade St.
Wadesboro, NC 28170
704-695-1000

Apria Healthcare Inc.
501 Covil Ave.
Wilmington, NC 28403
910-343-8930

Lincare
432 Landmark Dr.
Wilmington, NC 28412
910-392-9208

PSA Home Healthcare
2515 S. 17th St.
Wilmington, NC 28401
910-395-5266

American Home Patient
4421 N. Cherry St., # 30
Winston-Salem, NC 27105
336-767-7600

Lincare
2540 Viceroy Dr.
Winston-Salem, NC 27103
336-659-9021

OHIO

Apria Healthcare Inc.
1450 Firestone Pkwy.
Akron, OH 44301
330-773-2022

Apria Healthcare Inc.
8077 Leavitt Rd., # C
Amherst, OH 44001
440-986-2777

Lincare
1116 Lake Ave.
Ashtabula, OH 44004
440-964-6683

American Home Patient
1300 Clark St.
Cambridge, OH 43725
740-439-4848

American Home Patient
259 N. Woodbridge Ave.
Chillicothe, OH 45601
740-775-3544

Apria Healthcare Inc.
2327 Crowne Point Dr.
Cincinnati, OH 45241
513-772-1907

Caretenders
9280 Plainfield Rd.
Cincinnati, OH 45236
513-984-8000

Health Care Solutions
6161 Stewart Ave.
Cincinnati, OH 45227
513-271-5115

Homedco
2327 Crowne Point Dr.
Cincinnati, OH 45241
513-860-8710

Lincare
4329 Red Bank Rd.
Cincinnati, OH 45227
513-221-3050

Apria Healthcare Inc.
1000 Resource Dr.
Cleveland, OH 44131
216-485-1180

Caretenders
9885 Rockside Rd.
Cleveland, OH 44125
216-252-1558

Lincare
23130 Miles Rd.
Cleveland, OH 44128
216-328-0099

Lincare
18820 Bagley Rd., # 102
Cleveland, OH 44130
440-826-3104

NMC Homecare
6801 Engle Rd., # D
Cleveland, OH 44130
440-243-8900

Apria Healthcare Inc.
4060 Business Park Dr.
Columbus, OH 43204
614-351-5920

Caretenders
2000 Bethel Rd.
Columbus, OH 43220
614-457-1900

Apria Healthcare Inc.
7740 Washington Vill. Dr.
Dayton, OH 45459
937-438-1200

Lincare
3522 Encrete Lane
Dayton, OH 45439
937-299-1141

NMC Homecare
4406 Tuller Rd.
Dublin, OH 43017
614-889-2880

Apria Healthcare Inc.
1518 N. Main St., # 11
Lima, OH 45801
419-222-1500

Apria Healthcare Inc.
2151 Stumbo Rd.
Mansfield, OH 44906
419-529-8333

Lincare
2565 Harding Hwy E.
Marion, OH 43302
740-382-1611

Apria Healthcare Inc.
737 W. Liberty St.
Medina, OH 44256
330-725-8333

Lincare
1949 Tamarack Rd.
Newark, OH 43055
740-349-8236

Caretenders
363 E. High St.
Springfield, OH 45505
937-323-4716

Apria Healthcare Inc.
2110 W. Central Ave.
Toledo, OH 43606
419-472-8080

Apria Healthcare Inc.
1501 Monroe St.
Toledo, OH 43624
419-242-9923

Lincare
3550 Executive Pkwy.
Toledo, OH 43606
419-535-6924

Lincare
402 E. Wilson Bridge Rd.
Worthington, OH 43085
614-885-9666

Caretenders
25 Market St.
Youngstown, OH 44503
330-746-9206

Apria Healthcare Inc.
1933 Maple Ave.
Zanesville, OH 43701
740-452-0645

OKLAHOMA

American Home Patient
120 N. High St.
Antlers, OK 74523
580-298-3669

Lincare
830 Grand Ave.
Ardmore, OK 73401
580-226-7878

American Home Patient
100 S. Osage Ave.
Bartlesville, OK 74003
918-335-1100

Lincare
3327 E. Frank Phillips Blvd.
Bartlesville, OK 74006
918-333-4800

American Home Patient
200 W. Blue Starr Dr.
Claremore, OK 74017
918-341-7500

Lincare
553 S. 30th St.
Clinton, OK 73601
580-323-1377

Lincare
114 N. Oakwood Rd.
Enid, OK 73703
580-234-9922

American Home Patient
720 S. Main St.
Grove, OK 74344
918-786-1800

American Home Patient
6708 N.W. Cache Rd.
Lawton, OK 73505
580-536-3300

American Home Patient
223 E. Wyandotte Ave.
McAlester, OK 74501
918-426-1888

Apria Healthcare Inc.
6125 W. Reno Ave., # 300
Oklahoma City, OK 73127
405-495-1919

Lincare
4149 Highline Blvd.
Oklahoma City, OK 73108
405-947-0088

American Home Patient
Pawhuska, OK 74056
918-287-4100

Lincare
2115 Hwy. 9 W., # C
Seminole, OK 74868
405-382-2102

American Home Patient
5727 S. Garnett Rd.
Tulsa, OK 74146
918-250-0449

Apria Healthcare Inc.
9902 E. 43rd St., # F
Tulsa, OK 74146
918-665-2255

Lincare
5527 E. 41st St.
Tulsa, OK 74135
918-622-7895

American Home Patient
404 W. Cherokee St., # E
Wagoner, OK 74467
918-485-4553

OREGON

Lincare
1110 S. Commercial Way,
S.E.
Albany, OR 97321
541-928-0333

Lincare
1210 Marine Dr.
Astoria, OR 97103
503-325-6733

Lincare
2525 N.E. Twin Knolls Dr.
Bend, OR 97701
541-382-8303

Lincare
2705 Kinney Rd.
Coos Bay, OR 97420
541-269-0607

Apria Healthcare Inc.
330 N.W. Elks Dr., # B
Corvallis, OR 97330
541-758-8335

Lincare
2795 Anderson Ave.
Klamath Falls, OR 97603
541-882-2325

Lincare
1112 Adams Ave.
La Grande, OR 97850
541-963-3118

Lincare
613 Market St.
Medford, OR 97504
541-773-2211

Lincare
158 S.E. 1st St.
Newport, OR 97365
541-265-5559

Apria Healthcare Inc.
6040 N. Cutter Cir.
Portland, OR 97217
503-735-0200

Apria Healthcare Inc.
12407 N.E. Marx St.
Portland, OR 97230
503-255-5864

Lincare
2719 N. Hayden Island Dr.
Portland, OR 97217
503-283-4193

Lincare
3470 Pipebend Pl., N.E.
Salem, OR 97301
503-362-8122

Lincare
623 W. Centennial Blvd.
Springfield, OR 97477
541-741-8330

PENNSYLVANIA

Apria Healthcare Inc.
1544 E. Pleasant Valley
Blvd.
Altoona, PA 16602
814-942-4702

Apria Healthcare Inc.
2041 Ave. C, # 400
Bethlehem, PA 18017
610-266-6333

American Home Patient
66 Main St.
Bradford, PA 16701
814-368-5990

American Home Patient
298 Main St.
Brookville, PA 15825
814-849-5353

American Home Patient
322 S. Logan Blvd.
Burnham, PA 17009
717-248-6761

Apria Healthcare Inc.
245 Pittsburgh Rd., # 404
Butler, PA 16001
412-654-3636

Apria Healthcare Inc.
3552 Gettysburg Rd.
Camp Hill, PA 17011
717-761-4630

Apria Healthcare Inc.
250 Technology Dr.
Canonsburg, PA 15317
412-655-8228

American Home Patient
100 W. High St.
Carlisle, PA 17013
717-249-7073

American Home Patient
497 Lincoln Way, E.
Chambersburg, PA 17201
717-267-2002

American Home Patient
4934 Peach St.
Erie, PA 16509
814-864-4974

Apria Healthcare Inc.
2401 W. 12th St.
Erie, PA 16505
814-454-5995

American Home Patient
38 Bedford Square
Everett, PA 15537
814-623-2141

Apria Healthcare Inc.
800 Primos Ave.
Folcroft, PA 19032
610-586-2000

Apria Healthcare Inc.
1000 Carlisle St.
Hanover, PA 17331
717-637-8090

American Home Patient
409 S. 2nd St., # 1A
Harrisburg, PA 17104
717-238-9683

American Home Patient
1550 E. State St.
Hermitage, PA 16148
412-983-1302

American Home Patient
919 Franklin St.
Johnstown, PA 15905
814-269-3199

Apria Healthcare Inc.
530 S. Henderson Rd., # C
King of Prussia, PA 19406
610-962-0744

NMC Homecare
1017 W. 9th Ave., # A
King of Prussia, PA 19406
610-337-9267

Apria Healthcare Inc.
240 Harrisburg Ave.
Lancaster, PA 17603
717-397-8000

Specialized Med. Devices
300 Running Pump Rd.
Lancaster, PA 17603
717-392-8570

Apria Healthcare Inc.
Latrobe, PA 15650
412-537-4401

American Home Patient
Emilie Rd. & Woerner Ave.
Levittown, PA 19057
215-946-0940

American Home Patient
201 E. Main St.
Lock Haven, PA 17745
717-748-1005

American Home Patient
4 McCormick Rd.
McKees Rocks, PA 15136
412-331-7366

Apria Healthcare Inc.
2628 Mosside Blvd.
Monroeville, PA 15146
412-373-4762

American Home Patient
R.R. 7, Box 1008
Mt. Pleasant, PA 15666
412-547-2080

Lincare
3411 5th Ave.
North Versailles, PA 15137
412-751-8300

American Home Patient
228 Seneca St.
Oil City, PA 16301
814-676-8865

NMC Homecare
500 Business Ctr. Dr., # 505
Pittsburgh, PA 15205
412-788-1280

American Home Patient
521 Mauch Chunk St.
Pottsville, PA 17901
717-628-5311

Apria Health Care
2300 N. 5th St.
Reading, PA 19605
610-374-0507

American Home Patient
2 N. Market St.
Shamokin, PA 17872
717-648-1178

American Home Patient
273 Benner Pike
State College, PA 16801
814-234-9771

American Home Patient
Drake Mall
Titusville, PA 16354
814-827-4644

American Home Patient
4667 Somerton Rd., # G
Trevose, PA 19053
215-396-9009

Lincare
159 Morgantown St., # C
Uniontown, PA 15401
412-439-9696

American Home Patient
200 Liberty St.
Warren, PA 16365
814-726-0300

American Home Patient
1051 E. Main St., # 4
Waynesboro, PA 17268
717-762-8141

American Home Patient
1128 Greenhill Rd.
West Chester, PA 19380
610-918-7440

American Home Patient
2615 Joppa Rd.
York, PA 17403
717-741-5353

Apria Healthcare Inc.
1500 N. George St.
York, PA 17404
717-848-8000

SOUTH CAROLINA

Lincare
1920 Dunbar St.
Charleston, SC 29407
843-769-4431

American Home Patient
115 Atrium Way, # 200
Columbia, SC 29223
803-736-1575

American Home Patient
127 Corporate Ln.
Columbia, SC 29223
803-714-6544

Apria Healthcare Inc.
6904 Main St.
Columbia, SC 29203
803-786-6900

American Home Patient
1701 Hwy. 544
Conway, SC 29526
843-347-0711

American Home Patient
181 E. Evans St., # 11
Florence, SC 29506
843-664-2818

Lincare
1612 N. Limestone St.
Gaffney, SC 29340
864-487-4778

Apria Healthcare Inc.
600 Front St.
Georgetown, SC 29440
843-527-8842

American Home Patient
11 Park Place Ct.
Greenville, SC 29607
864-299-0123

Lincare
1186 S. Main St.
Greenwood, SC 29646
864-227-3211

Apria Healthcare Inc.
4405 Socastee Blvd.
Myrtle Beach, SC 29575
843-293-6961

PSA Home Healthcare
2117 Wilson Rd.
Newberry, SC 29108
803-276-7635

American Home Patient
2030 Harley St.
No. Charleston, SC 29406
843-554-9785

Apria Healthcare Inc.
3540 Oscar Johnson Dr.
No. Charleston, SC 29405
843-747-0341

Apria Healthcare Inc.
130 Venture Blvd., # 4
Spartanburg, SC 29306
864-855-4413

Lincare
263 Broad St.
Sumter, SC 29150
803-773-0387

American Home Patient
442 N. Duncan Bypass
Union, SC 29379
864-429-8880

Lincare
1053 Sunset Blvd.
West Columbia, SC 29169
803-796-0775

SOUTH DAKOTA

Apria Healthcare Inc.
821 Mount Rushmore Rd.
Rapid City, SD 57701
605-341-2273

Apria Healthcare Inc.
802 W. 11th St.
Sioux Falls, SD 57104
605-334-8418

Apria Healthcare Inc.
1410 North Ave.
Spearfish, SD 57783
605-642-3990

TENNESSEE

American Home Patient
5200 Maryland Way, # 400
Brentwood, TN 37027
615-221-8884

American Home Patient
5958 Shallowford Rd.
Chattanooga, TN 37421
423-899-2434

Apria Healthcare Inc.
113 E. 2nd St., # 100
Chattanooga, TN 37403
423-266-2273

American Home Patient
380 S. Lowe Ave., # D
Cookeville, TN 38501
931-526-5514

American Home Patient
4569 Rhea County Hwy.
Dayton, TN 37321
423-775-3619

Lincare
1395 Flowering Dogwood
Lane
Dyersburg, TN 38024
901-286-0116

Apria Healthcare Inc.
1217 S. Roane St.
Harriman, TN 37748
423-882-0340

American Home Patient
919 N. Parkway
Jackson, TN 38305
901-423-3646

Apria Healthcare Inc.
2975 U.S. Hwy. 45 Bypass
Jackson, TN 38305
901-668-7611

Lincare
678 W. Forest Ave.
Jackson, TN 38301
901-424-1262

Apria Healthcare Inc.
1075 Martha Glass Dr.
Jefferson City, TN 37760
423-475-8953

American Home Patient
507 Princeton Rd.
Johnson City, TN 37601
423-282-5764

American Home Patient
555 E. Main St.
Kingsport, TN 37660
423-247-4032

Apria Healthcare Inc.
2021 Brookside Ln.
Kingsport, TN 37660
423-247-4277

American Home Patient
9111 Cross Park Dr.
Knoxville, TN 37923
423-539-8214

Apria Healthcare Inc.
1701 Louisville Dr., # A
Knoxville, TN 37921
423-588-5396

Apria Healthcare Inc.
5256 E. Raines Rd.
Memphis, TN 38118
901-368-1200

Lincare
4830 Lamar Ave.
Memphis, TN 38118
901-365-6977

American Home Patient
1102 Dow St.
Murfreesboro, TN 37130
615-895-6074

Apria Healthcare Inc.
1865 Air Lane Dr.
Nashville, TN 37210
615-889-8006

American Home Patient
480 Park Blvd.
Rogersville, TN 37857
423-272-4019

American Home Patient
211 E. Bransford St.
Union City, TN 38261
901-885-6060

TEXAS

Lincare
182 S. Willis St.
Abilene, TX 79605
915-672-7030

Lincare
2021 Coulter Dr.
Amarillo, TX 79106
806-358-7769

Lincare
1521 N. Cooper St., # 200
Arlington, TX 76011
817-274-1716

American Home Patient
1105 W. 41st St.
Austin, TX 78756
512-451-4519

Apria Healthcare Inc.
8868 Research Blvd., # 107
Austin, TX 78758
512-451-5599

Lincare
4631 Airport Blvd., # 122
Austin, TX 78751
512-467-8769

NMC Homecare
2324 Ridgepoint Dr., # F
Austin, TX 78754
512-928-8005

American Home Patient
4800 Avenue F
Bay City, TX 77414
409-245-1668

Lincare
6950 College St.
Beaumont, TX 77707
409-866-3775

Apria Healthcare Inc.
501 Birdwell Ln., # 3
Big Spring, TX 79720
915-263-0202

American Home Patient
2410 Coggin Ave.
Brownwood, TX 76801
915-643-4222

American Home Patient
3500 W. Davis St., # 270
Conroe, TX 77304
409-756-6060

Lincare
3421 W. Davis St., # 150
Conroe, TX 77304
409-756-9664

American Home Patient
226 S. Enterprise Pkwy.
Corpus Christi, TX 78405
512-289-7177

Apria Healthcare Inc.
4310 Kostoryz Rd.
Corpus Christi, TX 78415
512-851-0671

Lincare
4455 S. Spid, # 30
Corpus Christi, TX 78411
512-814-1666

Lincare
701 W. 2nd Ave.
Corsicana, TX 75110
903-872-6503

American Home Patient
3950 Doniphan Park Cir.
El Paso, TX 79922
915-585-2112

Apria Healthcare Inc.
10737 Gateway Blvd. W.
El Paso, TX 79935
915-594-8203

Lincare
5360 N. Mesa St., # 112
El Paso, TX 79912
915-845-2000

American Home Patient
4609 Fairlane Ave.
Fort Worth, TX 76119
817-641-6600

Apria Healthcare Inc.
8300 Esters Blvd., # 920
Fort Worth, TX 76155
817-621-2005

Lincare
4822 Hwy. 377 S.
Fort Worth, TX 76116
817-560-4618

Lincare
1209 W.N. Carrier Pkwy.
Grand Prairie, TX 75050
972-988-1801

Lincare
1012 W. Main St., # 102
Gun Barrel City, TX 75147
903-887-5005

American Home Patient
501 N. Ed Carey Dr.
Harlingen, TX 78550
956-423-8385

Apria Healthcare Inc.
410 N. Ed Carey Dr., # A
Harlingen, TX 78550
956-428-4091

American Home Health
3802 Blodgett St.
Houston, TX 77004
713-521-0053

American Home Patient
9488 Kirby Dr.
Houston, TX 77054
713-660-0000

Apria Healthcare Inc.
5301 Hollister St.
Houston, TX 77040
713-588-5500

Apria Healthcare Inc.
1895 W. Sam Houston
Pkwy. N.
Houston, TX 77043
281-588-5550

Lincare
9030 Kirby Dr.
Houston, TX 77054
713-666-4500

NMC Homecare
900 S. Loop W.
Houston, TX 77054
713-747-5111

American Home Patient
306 S. Skyway Cir.
Irving, TX 75038
972-257-0988

American Home Patient
120 Hwy. 332
Lake Jackson, TX 77566
409-297-1823

American Home Patient
2333 E. Saunders St., # 3
Laredo, TX 78041
956-725-5066

American Home Patient
603 N. 2nd St.
Longview, TX 75601
903-758-7162

Lincare
821 N. 4th St.
Longview, TX 75601
903-234-2233

American Home Patient
3702 20th St., # A
Lubbock, TX 79410
806-792-9844

Apria Healthcare Inc.
4619 W. Loop 289
Lubbock, TX 79414
806-791-0202

American Home Patient
1120 Lindberg Ave., # 1
McAllen, TX 78501
956-631-5461

Lincare
508 N. 10th St.
McAllen, TX 78501
956-682-0911

Lincare
2414 W. University Dr.
McKinney, TX 75070
972-548-0007

American Home Patient
3205 N. University Dr., # I
Nacogdoches, TX 75961
409-564-5929

American Home Health
408 N. Washington Ave.
Odessa, TX 79761
915-580-4322

Apria Healthcare Inc.
1355 E. 8th St.
Odessa, TX 79761
915-335-0202

American Home Patient
1541 N. Hobart St.
Pampa, TX 79065
806-669-0000

American Home Patient
3404 Olton Rd., # C
Plainview, TX 79072
806-296-6433

American Home Patient
626 E. Market St.
Rockport, TX 78382
512-729-6993

American Home Patient
111 W. Twohig Ave.
San Angelo, TX 76903
915-942-6432

American Home Patient
4319 Med. Dr.
San Antonio, TX 78229
210-614-0110

Apria Healthcare Inc.
14220 Northbrook Dr.
San Antonio, TX 78232
210-494-0203

Lincare
7909 Fredericksburg Rd.
San Antonio, TX 78229
210-614-1118

NMC Homecare
12500 Network Blvd., # 210
San Antonio, TX 78249
210-561-8800

Apria Healthcare Inc.
217 N. Walnut St.
Sherman, TX 75090
903-893-7411

American Home Patient
4613 S. 13th Ave.
Temple, TX 76502
254-778-7131

Lincare
4148 S.W. H. K. Dodgen
Loop
Temple, TX 76504
254-774-8188

Lincare
3909 N. State Line Ave.
Texarkana, TX 75503
903-793-7776

Lincare
1861 Troup Hwy.
Tyler, TX 75701
903-595-6622

American Home Patient
2007 E. Red River St.
Victoria, TX 77901
512-573-0025

Lincare
5803 John Stockbauer Dr.
Victoria, TX 77904
512-578-0159

American Home Patient
3609 Bosque Blvd.
Waco, TX 76710
254-756-3202

Lincare
1501 Midwestern Pkwy.
Wichita Falls, TX 76302
940-723-9831

UTAH

Lincare
1550 Hill Field Rd.
Layton, UT 84041
801-825-4770

Interwest Home Med.
235 E. 6100 S.
Murray, UT 84107
801-261-5100

Lincare
46 N. 1200 W.
Orem, UT 84057
801-224-3338

Lincare
106 W. 2950 S.
Salt Lake City, UT 84115
801-487-0202

Whitmore Med.
1884 S. 300 W.
Salt Lake City, UT 84115
801-487-1065

Apria Healthcare Inc.
1555 W. 2200 S.
West Valley City, UT 84119
801-972-5353

VERMONT

Lincare
20 Technology Dr., # 6
Brattleboro, VT 5301
802-254-3880

Apria Healthcare Inc.
89 Ethan Allen Dr.
South Burlington, VT 5403
802-865-7801

VIRGINIA

Lincare
4200 Lafayette Ctr. Dr., # D
Chantilly, VA 20151
703-222-3090

Lincare
370 Greenbrier Dr., # D
Charlottesville, VA 22901
804-974-6688

American Home Patient
1700 S. Park Ct., # A
Chesapeake, VA 23320
757-523-5400

Apria Healthcare Inc.
814 Greenbrier Cir.
Chesapeake, VA 23320
757-420-1641

Lincare
816 Greenbrier Cir., # E
Chesapeake, VA 23320
757-424-4822

NMC Homecare
1800 Coyote Dr.
Chester, VA 23836
804-768-1200

American Home Patient
1131 S. Main St.
Farmville, VA 23901
804-392-1853

Lincare
120 E. Grayson St.
Galax, VA 24333
540-238-8880

Apria Healthcare Inc.
8210 Cinderbed Rd.
Lorton, VA 22079
703-550-8355

Apria Healthcare Inc.
317 Hospital Dr.
Martinsville, VA 24112
540-638-3353

American Home Patient
520 Southlake Blvd.
Richmond, VA 23236
804-278-9706

Apria Health Care
7401 Whitepine Rd.
Richmond, VA 23237
804-271-8171

Caretenders
2601 Willard Rd., # 101
Richmond, VA 23294
804-672-7500

Caretenders
1717 Bellevue Ave.
Richmond, VA 23227
804-264-9614

Lincare
4912 W. Marshall St.
Richmond, VA 23230
804-355-2323

Apria Healthcare Inc.
5151 Starkey Rd., # B
Roanoke, VA 24014
540-772-0411

American Home Patient
1790 Apperson Dr.
Salem, VA 24153
540-375-3152

Apria Healthcare Inc.
504 Shaw Rd.
Sterling, VA 20166
703-444-3322

Lincare
301 Cleveland Pl., # 101
Virginia Beach, VA 23462
757-671-1802

WASHINGTON

Lincare
400 E. Wishkah St.
Aberdeen, WA 98520
360-532-5287

Lincare
1501 15th St., N.W.
Auburn, WA 98001
253-833-6075

Apria Healthcare Inc.
470 Birchwood Ave.
Bellingham, WA 98225
360-738-8300

Lincare
801 W. Orchard Dr., # 8
Bellingham, WA 98225
360-671-3813

Apria Healthcare Inc.
5299 State Hwy. 303, N.E.
Bremerton, WA 98311
360-479-7164

Lincare
1058 N.W. State Ave.
Chehalis, WA 98532
360-748-4534

Lincare
615 Elm St.
Clarkston, WA 99403
509-758-5400

Lincare
44 Rock Island Rd.
East Wenatchee, WA 98802
509-884-0666

Lincare
5113 Pacific Hwy. E.
Fife, WA 98424
253-922-3137

Apria Healthcare Inc.
7919 W. Grandridge Blvd.
Kennewick, WA 99336
509-783-8413

Lincare
6515 W. Clearwater Ave.
Kennewick, WA 99336
509-783-1411

Lincare
5625 48th Dr., N.E.
Marysville, WA 98270
360-659-9823

Lincare
1401 E. Wheeler Rd.
Moses Lake, WA 98837
509-766-6038

Lincare
424 Lilly Rd., N.E.
Olympia, WA 98506
360-923-1985

Lincare
638 Okoma Dr.
Omak, WA 98841
509-826-5060

Lincare
1905 E. Front St.
Port Angeles, WA 98362
360-452-4724

Lincare
2421 Sims Way, # C
Port Townsend, WA 98368
360-385-1015

Apria Healthcare Inc.
14935 N.E. 87th St.
Redmond, WA 98052
425-881-8500

Lincare
9595 153rd Ave., N.E.
Redmond, WA 98052
425-869-8911

Lincare
1000 S.W. 7th St.
Renton, WA 98055
425-235-8186

Lincare
1101 N.W. Leary Way
Seattle, WA 98107
206-783-6444

Lincare
1245 4th Ave., S.
Seattle, WA 98134
206-467-8069

Lincare
3225 S. 116th St.
Seattle, WA 98168
206-241-1050

Apria Healthcare Inc.
820 S. McClellan St.
Spokane, WA 99204
509-456-8159

Apria Healthcare Inc.
411 E. North Foothills Dr.
Spokane, WA 99207
509-489-1000

Lincare
345 E. 3rd Ave.
Spokane, WA 99202
509-838-3888

Lincare
321 W. Hastings Rd.
Spokane, WA 99218
509-467-0362

Apria Healthcare Inc.
5102 20th St., E.
Tacoma, WA 98424
253-922-3200

PSA Home Healthcare
4201 N.E. 66th Ave., # 112
Vancouver, WA 98661
360-253-3744

Apria Healthcare Inc.
206 N. 6th Ave., # A
Yakima, WA 98902
509-452-1730

Lincare
20 N. 2nd St.
Yakima, WA 98901
509-248-7927

WEST VIRGINIA

Apria Healthcare Inc.
3202 Robert C. Byrd Dr.
Beckley, WV 25801
304-255-1464

Lincare
105 Platinum Dr., # C
Bridgeport, WV 26330
304-623-0622

Apria Healthcare Inc.
7003 Mountain Park Dr.
Fairmont, WV 26554
304-366-2874

Apria Healthcare Inc.
1941 3rd Ave.
Huntington, WV 25703
304-525-8585

Lincare
525 20th St.
Huntington, WV 25703
304-525-7238

NMC Homecare
1137 Van Voorhis Rd.
Morgantown, WV 26505
304-598-0515

Apria Healthcare Inc.
4210 1st Ave., # 310
Nitro, WV 25143
304-755-0718

Lincare
4200 1st Ave., # 112
Nitro, WV 25143
304-755-0431

Apria Healthcare Inc.
1170 46th St.
Parkersburg, WV 26101
304-295-0195

Apria Healthcare Inc.
22 National Rd.
Triadelphia, WV 26059
304-547-5555

WISCONSIN

Apria Healthcare Inc.
1316 N. Hastings Way, # B
Eau Claire, WI 54703
715-834-7517

American Home Patient
6330 Copps Ave.
Madison, WI 53716
608-222-5588

Apria Healthcare Inc.
434 S. Central Ave.
Marshfield, WI 54449
715-384-0088

American Home Patient
204 E. Upham St.
Marshfield, WI 54449
715-387-1789

Homedco
3315 N. 124th St.
Menomonee Falls, WI
53051
414-252-2400

American Home Patient
9442 N. 107th St.
Milwaukee, WI 53224
414-355-4561

American Home Patient
7342 Giles Dr.
Minocqua, WI 54548
715-356-2800

Apria Healthcare Inc.
859 E. Broadway
Monona, WI 53716
608-221-5480

Apria Healthcare Inc.
5345 S. Moorland Rd.
New Berlin, WI 53151
414-827-9100

Apria Healthcare Inc.
W6853 Industrial Blvd.
Onalaska, WI 54650
608-783-7668

American Home Patient
2725 Carlisle Ave.
Racine, WI 53404
414-633-7555

WYOMING

Lincare
545 Budd Ave.
Big Piney, WY 83113
307-276-5744

Apria Healthcare Inc.
1700 W. 1st St., # 3
Casper, WY 82604
307-577-0696

Lincare
1842 E. 2nd St.
Casper, WY 82601
307-237-8000

Lincare
3150 Energy Ln.
Casper, WY 82604
307-237-1004

Apria Healthcare Inc.
515 E. Carlson St.
Cheyenne, WY 82009
307-634-7121

Lincare
1221 E. Pershing Blvd.
Cheyenne, WY 82001
307-637-8267

Vital Air
502 Blackburn Ave.
Cody, WY 82414
307-587-4953

Lincare
117 N. 2nd St.
Douglas, WY 82633
307-358-5805

Lincare
120 Yellow Creek Rd.
Evanston, WY 82930
307-789-6621

Lincare
709 W. 8th St.
Gillette, WY 82716
307-687-0501

Vital Air
346 Greybull Ave.
Greybull, WY 82426
307-765-4406

Lincare
401 Garfield St.
Laramie, WY 82070
307-721-4992

Vital Air
184 E. Main
Lovell, WY 82431
307-548-2708

Lincare
1121 Washington Blvd., # 2
Newcastle, WY 82701
307-746-2281

Vital Air
233 E. 2nd St.
Powell, WY 82435
307-754-4524

Lincare
409 W. Cedar St.
Rawlins, WY 82301
307-324-2117

Lincare
702 E. Monroe Ave.
Riverton, WY 82501
307-856-7562

Lincare
2730 Commercial Way
Rock Springs, WY 82901
307-382-7703

Lincare
655 Broadway St.
Sheridan, WY 82801
307-672-0073

Lincare
228 N. 10th St.
Worland, WY 82401
307-347-2674

APPENDIX THREE

Sleep Disorders Dental Society Membership

This information was provided by the Sleep Disorders Dental Society. For additional information on dental procedures for snoring and sleep apnea, contact Mary Beth Rogers, Executive Director, Sleep Disorders Dental Society, 10592 Perry Highway, #220, Wexford, PA 15090-9244 (phone: 724-935-0836).

ALABAMA

Barnes III, Ernest M.
500 Whitesport Dr., # 2
Huntsville, AL 35801
256-883-5771

Blackmon, Keith A.
107 Professional Ln.
Dothan, AL 36303
334-792-5711

Doekel, Robert C.
Sleep Disorders Ctr.
of Alabama
790 Montclair Rd., # 200
Birmingham, AL 35213
205-599-1020

Langley, Barry L.
4720 Airport Blvd.
Mobile, AL 36608
334-344-4994

Morgan, Richard E.
2512-D Rocky Ridge Rd.
Birmingham, AL 35243
205-823-6733

Walker Jr., Joseph A.
630 Leighton Ave.
Anniston, AL 36207
256-236-1623

ALASKA

Chang, Ken Y.
9500 Independence Dr.
Anchorage, AK 99507
907-522-1685

ARIZONA

Bernstein, Allan K.
3030 N. 67th Place, # D
Scottsdale, AZ 85251
602-949-1234

Davis, Richard C.
2777 N. Campbell Ave.
Tucson, AZ 85719
520-795-9202

Davis, W. Morgan
1551 East University Dr.
Mesa, AZ 85203
602-834-6777

ARKANSAS

Harkins, Stephen J.
6367 E. Tangue Verde
Tucson, AZ 85715
520-298-6909

Hurd, Herman E.
500 S. University
Little Rock, AR 72205
501-664-0111

Janisse, Robert C.
702 E. Bell Rd., # 118
Phoenix, AZ 85022
602-404-3483

Phillips, David P.
2420 S. 51st Court
Fort Smith, AR 72903
501-452-2994

Remerscheid, Dale M.
400 N. Walton Blvd., # D
Bentonville, AR 72712
501-273-3800

Strong, Sam M.
1415 Breckenridge Dr.
Little Rock, AR 72227
501-224-2333

CALIFORNIA

Abramson, Mark E.
35 Renato Court
Redwood City, CA 94061
415-369-9227

Alvarez, R. Michael
2188 Peralta Blvd., # D
Fremont, CA 94536
510-713-6790

Armistead, Daniel B.
2233 Alma St.
Palo Alto, CA 94301
415-326-4466

Batcha, Debbie A.
1510 Park Ave., # 100
San Jose, CA 95126
408-293-1342

Berger, Joel S.
8008 Frost St., # 311
San Diego, CA 92123
619-292-5175

Berick, Joel D.
6529 Mission Gorge Rd.
San Diego, CA 92120
619-283-3161

Blum, Michael P.
1211 W. La Palma Ave.
Anaheim, CA 92801
714-772-2200

Botoaca, Dan C.
3200 La Crescenta Ave.
Glendale, CA 91208
818-541-9278

Chase, Douglas
20 Doctors Park Dr.
Santa Rosa, CA 95405
707-578-7701

Chase, Peter F.
Univ. of the Pacific Facial
Pain Ctr.
2155 Webster St., Rm. 615
San Francisco, CA 94115
415-929-6611

Clark, Glenn T.
10833 Le Conte Ave.
Box 951668, Rm. 43-009
Los Angeles, CA 90095
310-825-6406

Connolly, Francis B.
P.O. Box 1492
Shingle Springs, CA 95682
916-929-2676

Didier, Robert P.
2305 Mendocino Ave.
Santa Rosa, CA 95403
707-525-1560

Duhamel, James B.
1919 Vista Del Lago, # 4
Valley Springs, CA 95252
209-772-9649

Eckhart, James
321 12th St.
Manhattan Beach, CA
90266

Eich, William C.
1799 N. Waterman Ave.
San Bernardino, CA 92404
909-883-4226

Eli, Bradley A.
P.O. Box 234213
Encinitas, CA 92023
619-931-6555

Fenton, Douglas F.
One Embarcadero Ctr.
San Francisco, CA 94111
415-421-4772

George, Mark A.
1140 W. La Veta Ave., # 530
Orange, CA 92668
714-953-1000

Gereis, Mahfouz M.
8227 Van Nuys Blvd.
Panorama City, CA 91402
818-989-3074

Green, Robert E.
27292 Messina St., # A
Highland, CA 92346
909-862-2396

Growney Jr., Maurice R.
790 Ulloa St.
San Francisco, CA 94127
415-566-8500

Gussman, Frank P.
1447 Second St.
Santa Monica, CA 90401
310-393-0521

Hayashi, Randall T.
601 16th St.
Modesto, CA 95354
209-521-1661

Holman, Kenneth A.
52 Arch St., # 2
Redwood City, CA 94062
415-366-5758

Hoy, Jeffrey P.
3440 W. Lomita Blvd.
Torrance, CA 90505
310-326-7421

Inouye, Randall N.
162 Town & Country Vill.
Palo Alto, CA 94301
650-321-3266

Ivanhoe, John R.
School of Dentistry
Med. College of Georgia
Augusta, GA 30912
706-721-2554

Kigawa, Steve H.
12802 Washington Blvd.
Los Angeles, CA 90066
310-305-8404

Kim, Dosung
220-B Standiford Ave.
Modesto, CA 95350
209-526-4244

Kramer, Bernard M.
3838 California St., # 504
San Francisco, CA 94118
415-221-5512

Kremen, Gin P.
552 N. Franklin St.
Fort Bragg, CA 95437
707-964-6489

Lackey, Arlen D.
675 Pine Ave.
Pacific Grove, CA 93950
831-649-1055

Larson, Kirk B.
100 East Valencia Mesa Dr.
Fullerton, CA 92835
714-870-9445

Latham, Gary M.
5029 Deerwood Dr.
Santa Rosa, CA 95401
707-527-7400

Laver, Thomas J.
11376 Pleasant Valley Rd.
Penn Valley, CA 95946
530-432-5497

Lee, Raymond
4522 Indianola Way
La Canada, CA 91011
818-790-2778

Marshall, Michael W.
14343 Bellflower Blvd.
Bellflower, CA 90706
310-866-3727

Matsumura, Wynn
3030 Geary Blvd.
San Francisco, CA 94118
415-387-8600

McGwire, John T.
350 Vinton Ave., # 102
Pomona, CA 91767
909-620-1913

Mickiewicz, Timothy E.
2801 Capitol Ave., # 210
Sacramento, CA 95816
916-457-7710

Miller, David B.
2648 Del Paso Blvd.
Sacramento, CA 95815
916-925-2264

Moe, Larry A.
20899A Spanish Grant Dr.
Sonora, CA 95370
209-533-2225

Montgomery, Michael C.
8055 W. Manchester Ave.
Playa Del Rey, CA 90293
310-821-0992

Morgan, Todd D.
320 Sante Fe Dr., # 105
Encinitas, CA 92024
619-436-9292

Newhart, Scott G.
416 N. Bedford Dr., # 311
Beverly Hills, CA 90210
310-550-1533

Okmin, Larry A.
10425 Tierrasanta Blvd.
San Diego, CA 92124
619-560-6374

Olmos, Steven R.
7811 La Mesa Blvd., # C
La Mesa, CA 91941
619-589-6060

Ortner Jr., Gerard T.
3001 P St.
Sacramento, CA 95816
916-736-6750

Pendegraft, Karl J.
5415 W. Hillsdale
Visalia, CA 93291
209-733-1097

Pitts, Walter C.
Sleep Ctr.,
Huntington Mem.
100 W. California
Pasadena, CA 91105
818-397-3061

Plessas, David J.
417 William St.
Vacaville, CA 95688
707-447-1700

Poss, Robert N.
343 Gellert Blvd., # D
Daly City, CA 94015
650-755-1222

Prinsell, Jeffrey R.
1950 Spectrum Cir.
Marietta, GA 30067
770-956-9856

Ramsey, Mary Lou
3351 El Camino Real, # 222
Atherton, CA 94027
415-299-9999

Reznick, Jay B.
5363 Balboa Blvd., # 233
Encino, CA 91316
818-788-4424

Riley, Roger E.
400 Newport Ctr. Dr.
Newport Beach, CA 92660
714-760-3883

Rutherford, Frederick C.
6200 Wilshire Blvd., # 1010
Los Angeles, CA 90048
323-937-0450

Saffold, Stephen P.
925 Secret River Dr.
Sacramento, CA 95831
916-391-2888

Saito, Edward T.
696 E. Colorado Blvd.
Pasadena, CA 91101
818-795-7877

Samaan, Wasseem A.
215 N. Harbor Blvd.
Fullerton, CA 92632
714-680-6767

Singer, Martin C.
1933 W. Valley Blvd.
Alhambra, CA 91803
626-289-6311

Smith, Rick K.
8030 Soquel Ave., # 101
Santa Cruz, CA 95062
408-462-5600

Swancutt, Max
1901 Westcliff Dr., # 4
Newport Beach, CA 92660
714-646-1120

Veis, Rob
9129 Lurline Ave.
Chatsworth, CA 91311
818-998-7460

Westbrook, Philip R.
104 E. Olive Ave., # 104
Redlands, CA 92373
909-793-9190

Wolf III, Charles
918 The Alameda
Berkeley, CA 94707
510-526-8813

Wolk, Roger S.
28 Malibu Colony Dr.
Malibu, CA 90265
310-456-6972

COLORADO

Bailey, Dennis R.
8925 S. Ridgeline Blvd.
Highlands Ranch, CO
80126
303-471-0044

Kennedy, James M.
3929 E. Arapahoe Rd.
Littleton, CO 80121
303-773-3695

Kneller, Timothy D.
12101 E. Iliff, # U
Aurora, CO 80014
303-696-9364

O'Brien, Richard F.
4500 E. 9th Ave., # 740
Denver, CO 80220
303-320-1221

Payne, Wayne F.
1619 N. Greenwood, # 102
Pueblo, CO 81003
719-542-4546

Pickle, B. Todd
4585 Hilton Pkwy., # 101
Colorado Spgs, CO 80907
719-599-0670

Savory, Gerald B.
5400 Mt. Meeker Rd.
Boulder, CO 80301
303-530-4145

Wilk, Steven J.
3540 S. Poplar St., # 301
Denver, CO 80237
303-758-4865

Winber, Stephen M.
1660 S. Albion St., # 1008
Denver, CO 80222
303-691-0267

CONNECTICUT

Brandler, Steven H.
890 Ethan Allen Hwy.
Ridgefield, CT 06877
203-438-7114

Cahn, Jeffrey
1435 Bedford St.
Stamford, CT 06905
203-323-2882

Chassanoff, Arnold L.
87 Slater Ave.
Jewett City, CT 06351
203-376-9855

Demas, Donald C.
453 Main St.
Watertown, CT 06795
860-274-6625

Greenwald, Michael M.
160 Robbins St.
Waterbury, CT 06708
203-757-8855

Schwaber, David P.
P.O. Box 2003
Burlington, CT 06013
860-673-9141

Yanell, Donald D.
83 East Ave., # 202
Norwalk, CT 06851
203-838-2003

Zitnay, Johna D.
4949 Main St.
Stratford, CT 06611
203-375-7749

WASHINGTON, DC

Loube, Daniel I.
Sleep Disorders Ctr.,
Pulmonary SVC
Walter Reed Army Med. Ctr.
Washington, DC 20307
202-782-5724

Peterson, Larry J.
1234 19th St. N.W., # 200
Washington, DC 20036
202-785-0555

FLORIDA

Baumbauer, Jon M.
240 Pine St.
Homosasstt, FL 34446
904-746-0330

Corn, Jack H.
3400 Bee Ridge Rd., # 100
Sarasota, FL 34239
941-924-4210

Craig, John E.
815 Wicklow Court
Orange Park, FL 32065
904-276-5945

Dann III, Carl
2200 E. Robinson St.
Orlando, FL 32803
407-894-3271

Esser, David C.
1590 N.W. 10th Ave., # 302
Boca Raton, FL 33486
407-392-4303

Freedline, Randy D.
20911 N.W. 2nd Ave.
Miami, FL 33169
305-651-7676

Goldberg, Howell A.
815 S. University Dr., #102
Plantation, FL 33324
954-472-3303

Hernandez Jr., Nilo A.
8740 N. Kendall Dr.
Miami, FL 33176
305-279-1643

King, Roy K.
24 Loxahatchee Dr., # 4
Jupiter, FL 33458
407-747-5766

Langston, Gregory G.
165 Fifth Ave., N.E.
St. Petersburg, FL 33701
813-823-1993

Lawton, Thomas C.
201 N. Lakemont Ave.
Winter Park, FL 32792
407-644-8242

Martell, Bayardo
P.O. Box 526150
Miami, FL 33152
502-339-2863

Morrish Jr., James A.
708 43rd St.
Bradenton, FL 34209
941-746-2463

O'Leary, Kay W.
2286 Tamiami Trail
Port Charlotte, FL 33952
941-627-2011

Shipman, Barry
Oral Surgery, # 2089
1475 N.W. 12th Ave.
Miami, FL 33136
305-243-9390

GEORGIA

Black, Harold A.
908 E. 66th St.
Savannah, GA 31405
912-355-5000

Finkel, Robert A.
Gwinnett Place Commons
3796 Satellite Blvd., # 100
Duluth, GA 30136
770-497-9111

Haywood, Van B.
Dept. of Oral Rehabilitation
Med. College of GA
Augusta, GA 30912
706-721-2554

O'Connor, Frank L.
2258 Northlake Pkwy.
Tucker, GA 30084
770-939-5661

Tilley, Larry L.
508 S. Wall St.
Calhoun, GA 30701
706-629-0131

HAWAII

George, Peter T.
1649 Kalakaua Ave.
Honolulu, HI 96826
808-946-9658

IDAHO

Gaffner, Vernon O.
333 S. Woodruff Ave.
Idaho Falls, ID 83401
208-524-2034

Spencer, Jamison R.
2030 N. Cole Rd.
Boise, ID 83704
208-376-3600

Wright, Mark W.
1415 N. Fillmore, # 701
Twin Falls, ID 83301
208-735-1415

ILLINOIS

Antonakos, Anargyros S.
1637 Waukegan Rd.
Glenview, IL 60025
847-657-0750

Di Verde, Richard B.
30 S. Michigan Ave., # 300
Chicago, IL 60603
312-263-7822

Krueger, Michael J.
12 E. Miller Rd.
Sterling, IL 61081
815-625-0053

Kurtz, Glenn A.
411 Beck Rd.
Lindenhurst, IL 60046
847-356-3553

Liberati, Salvator P.
7606 McHenry Ave.
Crystal Lake, IL 60014
815-459-7800

Link, Mark R.
1027 S. Second
Springfield, IL 62704
217-522-4451

Milin, Kenneth N.
732 Elm St.
Winnetka, IL 60093
708-446-5868

Razdolsky, Yan
600 Lake Cook Rd., # 150
Buffalo Grove, IL 60089
847-215-7554

Rosen, Mark A.
Periodontics Ltd.
4711 Golf Rd., # 101
Skokie, IL 60076
847-675-7555

Rydstrom, Roger T.
333 W. First St.
Elmhurst, IL 60126
708-833-5110

Schwartz, David B.
9933 Lawler Ave.
Skokie, IL 60077
847-677-2808

Shapira, Ira L.
1810 Delany Rd.
Gurnee, IL 60031
847-623-5530

Sharifi, M. Nader
55 East Washington, # 3303
Chicago, IL 60602
312-236-1576

Wilmert, W. James
113 Pine St.
Lincoln, IL 62656
217-732-8523

Woodside, Honore
9933 Lawler, # 417
Skokie, IL 60077
847-329-0464

INDIANA

Akard, Sarah
3715 Kentucky Ave., # B
Indianapolis, IN 46221
317-856-2309

Bagnoli, Michael L.
2020 Union St., # 200
Earlhurst Professional Bldg.
Lafayette, IN 47904
765-446-8808

Bojrab, David G.
4606-D East State St.
Ft. Wayne, IN 46815
219-423-2340

Ingleman, Jon D.
223 E. Tillman Rd.
Fort Wayne, IN 46816
219-447-2568

Magnetti, Thomas R.
2646 Lois St.
Portage, IN 46368
219-762-4266

Smith, Harold A.
5435 Emerson Way N.
Indianapolis, IN 46226
317-547-0045

IOWA

Bender, Stephen T.
107 S. Pine
Bloomfield, IA 52537
515-665-1121

Elsner, Katherine
4626 University Ave.
Des Moines, IA 50311
515-277-3766

McManis, Mary Schilling
828 N. 7th
Burlington, IA 52601
319-752-8142

Walgren, James C.
1122 Rockdale Rd.
Dubuque, IA 52003
319-556-2650

KANSAS

Dowling, David F.
11644 W. 75th, # 101
Shawnee Mission, KS 66214
913-268-7077

Speake, Bruce A.
2887 S.W. Mac Vicar Ave.
Topeka, KS 66611
913-267-6301

KENTUCKY

Falace, Donald A.
U. of Kentucky College
of Denistry
Oral Diagnosis/Oral
Medicine
Lexington, KY 40536
606-323-5279

Kuhl, Robert W.
13001 U.S. Hwy. 42
Prospect, KY 40059
502-228-6100

McCrillis, John M.
3500 Bardstown Rd.
Louisville, KY 40218
502-458-7476

Mettens, Donn E.
1807 Alexandria Pike
Highland Hts, KY 41076
606-781-7200

Ney, Marshall J.
527 W. Main St.
Richmond, KY 40476
606-623-3761

LOUISIANA

Hollembeak, Perry W.
2001 E. 70th St., # 108
Shreveport, LA 71105
318-797-3362

Verdun, Larry J.
1001-B East 7th St.
Thibodaux, LA 70301
504-446-8474

MAINE

Armstrong, Daniel J.
192 Western Ave.
South Portland, ME 04106
207-773-1703

Battel, Cynthia A.
280 Commercial St.
Rockport, ME 04856
207-236-6675

Estabrooks, Lewis N.
20 Long Creek Dr.
So. Portland, ME 04106
207-772-4063

Fairbanks, Carlton E.
20 Long Creek Dr.
So. Portland, ME 04106
207-772-4063

MARYLAND

Anolik, Steven M.
19221 Montgomery
Village Ave.
Montgomery Village, MD
20886
301-948-8838

Hall, Armand
12714 Ocean Gateway
Ocean City, MD 21842
410-213-1010

Lever, Scott A.
20 Crossroads Dr., # 110
Owings Mills, MD 21117
410-363-2500

Mintz, Sylvan S.
6192 Oxon Hill Rd., # 601
Oxon Hill, MD 20745
301-839-1330

Schindler, Irv H.
8640 Guilford Rd., # 221A
Columbia, MD 21046
410-381-7300

Singer, Michael T.
10215 Fernwood Rd.
Bethesda, MD 20817
301-493-9500

Tilkin, Robert B.
11301 Rockville Pike
3rd Level White Flint
North Bethesda, MD 20895
301-881-6170

MASSACHUSETTS

Cohen, Robert B.
Harvard School of Dental
Medicine
188 Longwood Ave.
Boston, MA 02115
617-432-2374

Demko, B. Gail
P.O. Box 610230
Newton Highlands, MA
02161
617-964-4028

Katz, Matthew
1795 Main St.
Springfield, MA 01103
413-732-7208

Komyati, Stephen E.
HPHC/Dental Unit
Two Fenway Plaza
Boston, MA 02215
617-421-1122

Lake Jr., John R.
3854 Falmouth Rd.
Marstons Mills, MA 02648
508-428-4929

Lockerman, Larry Z.
U. Mass Mem. Med. Ctr.
119 Belmont St.
Worcester, MA 01605
860-528-3427

Mehta, Noshir R.
One Kneeland St.
Boston, MA 02111
617-636-6817

Satloff, David
44 Whiting St.
North Attleboro, MA 02760
508-695-1078

Yolin, Herbert S.
1842 Beacon St.
Brookline, MA 02146
617-730-8989

MICHIGAN

Ash, Major M.
Univ. of Michigan
School of Dentistry
Ann Arbor, MI 48109
313-647-4296

Ashman, Lawrence M.
32931 Middlebelt Rd.
Farmington Hills, MI 48334
810-737-7950

Bartoszek, Edward J.
902 S. Euclid Ave.
Bay City, MI 48706
517-684-0873

Drozdowicz, Martin A.
5323 Raven Pkwy.
Monroe, MI 48161
313-243-6282

Flood, Kevin P.
4990 Cascade, S.E.
Grand Rapids, MI 49546
616-974-4990

Fortson, Raymond A.
35200 Schoolcraft
Livonia, MI 48150
734-261-8860

Geb, Ronald D.
39960 Garfield
Clinton Twp., MI 48038
810-286-8530

Girard, Charles J.
2027 Fourth St.
Jackson, MI 49203
517-787-9630

Hanna, Charles E.
1504 Harcrest
Midland, MI 48640
517-631-2900

Heeke, David W.
2410 Lake Lansing Rd.
Lansing, MI 48912
517-484-4455

Hollister, Steven E.
209 East Mason
Owosso, MI 48867
517-725-7505

Kaspo, Ghabi A.
2959 Crooks Rd., # 7
Troy, MI 48084
248-649-6610

Lamoreaux, Edward L.
2424 Spring Arbor Rd.
Jackson, MI 49203
517-787-2226

Lesser, Morton B.
6425 Apple Grove Lane
Bloomfield Hills, MI 48301
248-851-8511

Mansour, Nizar N.
28035 Southfield Rd.
Lathrup Village, MI 48076
248-559-9110

Marion, Ronald P.
22190 Garrison, # 205
Dearborn, MI 48124
313-562-3388

Palumbo, Charles H.
601 S. Shore Dr., # 225
Battle Creek, MI 49015
616-964-7557

Rouff, Douglas M.
31700 W. 12 Mile, # 103
Farmington Hills, MI 48334
810-553-4660

Scavo, Richard F.
31158 Haggerty
Farmington Hills, MI 48331
248-661-5900

Smoler, Bruce A.
820 N. Wayne Rd.
Westland, MI 48185
313-728-5600

Sturtz, David H.
9416 S. Main St.
Plymouth, MI 48170
313-455-0710

Tatro, Richard J.
2123 N. Aurelius Rd.
Holt, MI 48842
517-699-2985

Totte, Tymon C.
18342 Mack Ave.
Grosse Pointe Farms, MI
48236
313-886-9201

Van Hook, Jeffery A.
37380 Glenwood
Westland, MI 48186
313-722-5130

Vanlandschoot, James P.
760 W. Washington St.
Marquette, MI 49855
906-228-4646

Zwetchkenbaum, Samuel
1011 N. University Ave.
Ann Arbor, MI 48109
313-936-6884

MINNESOTA

Bentley, Geoffrey D.
500 6th St.
Hawley, MN 56549
218-483-3311

Hakala, Roy V.
1690 University Ave., W.
St. Paul, MN 55104
612-642-1013

Kohler, Karen A.
6545 France Ave., S.
Edina, MN 55435
612-926-3858

Marshall, Todd W.
6545 France Ave., S.
Edina, MN 55435
612-926-3858

Parker, Jonathan A.
6600 Excelsior Blvd., # 191
Saint Louis Park, MN
55426
612-931-3176

Sanford, Richard A.
405 Sibley St., # 240
St. Paul, MN 55101
612-224-6824

MISSOURI

Cummings, Bruce C.
4444 N. Belleview, # 200
Gladstone, MO 64116
816-454-9090

Levy, Robert A.
777 S. New Ballas, # 206
St. Louis, MO 63141
314-569-0106

Myers, Terry L.
650 East 25th St.
Kansas City, MO 64108
816-235-2164

Palmer, Brian
4400 Broadway, # 514
Kansas City, MO 64111
816-561-5578

Wallace, Kevin D.
1200 E. Woodhurst, A-200
Springfield, MO 65804
417-881-1123

MONTANA

Casagrande, David W.
2105 Central Ave., # 100
Billings, MT 59102
406-656-2000

Melton, Sean F.
301 Saddle Dr.
Helena, MT 59601
406-443-1419

Meng, Vince W.
2831 Fort Missoula Rd.
Missoula, MT 59801
406-543-5647

Zlock, Gregory A.
Tribal Health
Mission Dr.
St. Ignatius, MT 59865
406-745-2411

NEBRASKA

Attanasio, Ronald
8232 Dorset Dr.
Lincoln, NE 68510
402-472-8820

Kutler, Benton
4239 Farnam St.
321 Doctors Bldg.
Omaha, NE 68131
402-552-2800

Miller, Thomas E.
702 S. Bailey
North Platte, NE 69101
308-532-1911

Sheridan, Paul J.
600 S. 42nd St.
Omaha, NE 68198
402-559-9200

NEVADA

Ahlstrom, Robert H.
3701 Baker Lane, # 2
Reno, NV 89509
702-827-8080

D'ascoli, Vincent P.
1407 N. Carson St.
Carson City, NV 89701
702-882-1062

Kennedy, Barry A.
4818 W. Lone Mntn. Rd.
Las Vegas, NV 89130
702-655-9533

NEW HAMPSHIRE

McKinney, Timothy L.
169 S. River Rd.
Bedford, NH 03110
607-625-6456

NEW JERSEY

Barbieri, Dennis
605 Broad Ave., # 101
Ridgefield, NJ 07657
201-941-9494

Belfer, William A.
804 W. Park Ave.
Ocean, NJ 07712
908-493-4747

Bershtein, Donald B.
125 Livingston Ave.
Edison, NJ 08820
732-549-4974

Blumenstock, Norman T.
410 Spotswood Englishtown Rd.
Spotswood, NJ 08884
732-251-7766

Ciuffreda, Leonard R.
900 W. Main St.
Freehold, NJ 07728
908-303-6000

Cohen, Stephen R.
1793 Springdale Rd.
Cherry Hill, NJ 08003
609-424-7177

Crain, Janet
Tor Plaza 35
2045 Route 35 South
So. Amboy, NJ 08879
908-727-5000

Elassar, Michael
501 Bloomfield Ave., # 2E
Caldwell, NJ 07006
201-228-1333

Flinn Jr., Clair William
150 N. Finley Ave.
Basking Ridge, NJ 07920
908-766-0111

Friedman, Robert S.
39 E. Hanover Ave.
Morris Plains, NJ 07950
973-539-0708

Fu, Tzulin T.
186 A Smith St.
Perth Amboy, NJ 08861
732-442-6000

Geron, Philip R.
Westfield Oral Surgery
320 Lenox Ave.
Westfield, NJ 07090
908-233-8088

Grossman, Harry P.
2864 Route 27, # B
North Brunswick, NJ 08902
732-297-6111

Harris, Robert J.
141 Terrace St.
Haworth, NJ 07641
201-384-1717

Haze, John J.
150 River Rd.
Montville, NJ 07045
201-263-9190

Hilsen, Kenneth L.
555 North Ave.
Fort Lee, NJ 07024
201-592-1818

Hutchings, Michael L.
14 Manor Dr.
Mt. Holly, NJ 08060
609-724-3787

Kadish, Abraham J.
1395 Route 23
Kinnelon / Butler, NJ 07405
201-492-8100

Katz, Michael
607 Station Ave.
Haddon Heights, NJ 08035
609-547-9151

Kazella, Ignatius J.
5 Sicomac Rd.
North Haledon, NJ 07508
201-423-3399

Krinks, Gregory J.
125 W. Broad St.
Paulsboro, NJ 08066
609-423-0716

Kulak, Chester B.
2796 Princeton Pike
Lawrenceville, NJ 08648
609-882-9443

Lavacca, Anthony
166 Franklin Ave.
Ridgewood, NJ 07450
201-652-2474

Legband, Frederick T.
420 Blvd., # 102
Mountain Lakes, NJ 07046
973-263-2770

Levine, Jerome H.
256 Columbia Tpke., # 107
Florham Park, NJ 07932
973-822-1200

Levitt, Richard E.
1815 New Rd.
Northfield, NJ 08225
609-646-0333

Messing, Michael G.
68 Essex St.
Millburn, NJ 07041
973-992-4770

Miranti, Richard A.
1201 Hwy. 37 E.
Toms River, NJ 08753
908-929-2250

Morton, M. Jeffrey
232 Chester Ave.
Moorestown, NJ 08057
609-778-1666

Pereira, Benjamin
1315 Anderson Ave.
Fort Lee, NJ 07024
201-943-1333

Pisano, Dominic D.
797 Springfield Ave.
Summit, NJ 07901
908-273-1525

Rosen, Ira S.
2186 State Hwy. 27
North Brunswick, NJ 08902
732-422-7440

Rosenbloom, Donald T.
18 Halco Dr.
Paramus, NJ 07652
201-262-8369

Samani, Mark F.
555 North Ave.
Fort Lee, NJ 07024
201-592-1818

Soldinger, Barry H.
220 Union Mill Rd.
Mt. Laurel, NJ 08054
609-778-0022

Stark, Thomas
1323 Hwy. 27
Somerset, NJ 08873
908-249-3350

Ueda, Taiji
1565 Palisade Ave.
Fort Lee, NJ 07024
201-461-0003

Winter, Fred J.
1 Elm Court
Metuchen, NJ 08840
908-548-4172

NEW MEXICO

Meade, Thomas E.
3748 Eubank, N.E.
Albuquerque, NM 87111
505-299-9172

NEW YORK

Barsh, Laurence I.
30 W. 61st St., # 11 D
New York, NY 10023
212-315-0913

Bernstein, Ira M.
9 Johnsons Lane
New City, NY 10956
914-634-0021

Binder, David S.
745 Fifth Ave., # 1405
New York, NY 10151
212-753-0500

Campo, Gerald F.
189 Stone Ridge Dr.
Rochester, NY 14615
716-621-6460

Chernick, Alan J.
Esquire Professional Bldg.
10 Esquire Rd.
New City, NY 10956
914-638-4880

Danziger, Fred
324 W. Park Ave.
Long Beach, NY 11561
516-432-2837

Dibella, Jerome F.
189 Route 304
Pearl River, NY 10965
914-735-5111

Drew, Stephanie J.
2001 Marcus Ave., # N10
Lake Success, NY 11042
516-775-1818

Efron, Meryl J.
1145 Targee St.
Staten Island, NY 10304
718-667-4800

Elias, Arthur C.
101 East 79 St.
New York, NY 10021
212-737-2990

Faustini, Frederick R.
597 Route 22
Croton Falls, NY 10519
914-277-3919

Fischler, Arnold J.
242-02 61st Ave.
Douglaston, NY 11362
718-631-3030

Fisher, Robert L.
1 Rockefeller Plaza
New York, NY 10020
212-218-6699

Gelb, Michael L.
635 Madison Ave., Fl. 19
New York, NY 10022
212-752-1661

Greenberg, Gary S.
1700 State Tower Bldg.
Syracuse, NY 13202
315-422-1788

Gupta, Anant R.
P.O. Box 721165
Jackson Heights, NY 11372
718-533-1243

Howels, Jeffrey C.
St. Clare's Hosp.
Dept. of Dentistry
600 McClellan St.
Schenectady, NY 12304
518-382-2000 X5268

Hyde, Matthew
25-15 Bridge Plaza N., # 8
Long Island City, NY 11101
718-784-1741

Kaufman, Richard S.
2940 Lincoln Ave.
Oceanside, NY 11572
516-764-4224

Kesselschmidt, David
70 Glen Cove Rd.
Roslyn Heights, NY 11577
516-621-3777

Krueger, Gary D.
4796 Main St.
Snyder, NY 14226
716-839-5886

Laniado, Nadia
Harwood Bldg., # 312
Scarsdale, NY 10583
914-472-9595

Lichtenstein, Robert
420 Lexington Ave., # 228
New York, NY 10170
212-682-7200

Miller, Donald
200-17 Linden Blvd.
St. Albans, NY 11412
718-712-0605

Pantino, Don A.
309 Main St.
Islip, NY 11751
516-581-7777

Rein, Jeffrey S.
101 Hillside Ave., # A
Williston Park, NY 11596
516-741-6202

Seltzer, Neal
101 Hillside Ave., # A
Williston Park, NY 11596
516-741-6202

Sher, Martin R.
2215 Hendrickson St.
Brooklyn, NY 11234
718-252-4400

Sheren, Kevin L.
107 W. Main St.
East Islip, NY 11730
516-581-1188

Slavin, Mark R.
2534 Genesee St.
Utica, NY 13502
315-724-5141

Syrop, Steven B.
630 Fifth Ave., # 1857
New York, NY 10111
212-969-9166

Tanenbaum, Donald R.
630 5th Ave., # 1857
New York, NY 10111
212-265-0110

Tiso, Carmine L.
9530 Main St.
Clarence, NY 14031
716-759-2255

Wechterman, Ira P.
260 Middle Country Rd.
Selden, NY 11784
516-698-1140

Werner, Sheldon H.
111 Freedom Plains Rd.
Poughkeepsie, NY 12603
914-452-1770

Yun, Chongsun T.
400 Madison Ave.
New York, NY 10017
212-688-0320

Zweifler, Martin S.
80 Washington St.
Poughkeepsie, NY 12601
914-452-8550

NORTH CAROLINA

Clapp, Hubert B.
2912 Maplewood Ave.
Winston-Salem, NC 27103
910-765-8940

Moore, Kent E.
Presbyterian Med. Tower
1718 E. Fourth St.
Charlotte, NC 28204
704-358-8898

Norwood, W. Thomas
311 S. Main St.
Norwood, NC 28128
704-474-3152

Rider, Ernest A.
3535 Randolph Rd.
Charlotte, NC 28211
704-366-8936

Scurria, Mark S.
Dept. of Prosthodontics
UNC School of Dentistry
CB #7450
Chapel Hill, NC 27599
919-966-2712

NORTH DAKOTA

Deeter, Terry C.
1003 Gateway Ave.
Bismarck, ND 58501
701-222-1800

Fettig, Richard H.
311 N. Mandan St.
Bismarck, ND 58501
701-255-3130

OHIO

Brunetti, Donald J.
5671 Mahoning
Youngstown, OH 44515
216-793-9368

Danzeisen, Milo L.
4124 Shamley Green
Toledo, OH 43623
419-841-9570

Della Bella, Alexander M.
7835 Remington Road
Cincinnati, OH 45242
513-793-1977

Dormire, Richard H.
44 S. Main St.
Centerville, OH 45458
513-433-7166

Gay Jr., Walter E.
602 Main St., # 315
Cincinnati, OH 45202
513-381-7900

Hinkle, Robert M.
250 W. Bridge St.
Dublin, OH 43017
614-889-0777

Robins, Gary S.
8066 Hetz Dr.
Cincinnati, OH 45242
513-489-8344

Sreshta, Flavia P.
Dental Care at Marymount
12000 McCracken Rd.
Garfield Heights, OH 44125
216-663-1090

Venizelos, Christina G.
29101 Health Campus Dr.
Westlake, OH 44145
404-835-6220

OKLAHOMA

Cobble, Jan L.
8908 S. Yale, # 430
Tulsa, OK 74137
918-496-2481

Mongrain, Robert B.
7705 E. 81st St.
Tulsa, OK 74133
918-250-9528

Smith Jr., William P.
5120 S.E. Frank Phillips
Blvd.
Bartlesville, OK 74006
918-333-6300

OREGON

Beget, Barry C.
622 East 22nd Ave.
Eugene, OR 97405
541-687-2442

Royse, Norman E.
403 N.E. Franklin
Bend, OR 97701
503-382-6822

Simpson, Nicklis C.
220 N.W. John St.
Waldport, OR 97394
541-563-3945

PENNSYLVANIA

Berson, Evan Lyle
301 City Line Ave.
Bala Cynwyd, PA 19004
610-667-6666

Bresner, Michael I.
100 Pennsylvania Ave.
Irwin, PA 15642
412-864-1017

Dattilo, David J.
1501 Locust St.
Pittsburgh, PA 15219
412-281-3988

Fatica, Lawrence J.
2702 Zuck Rd.
Erie, PA 16506
814-833-3535

Fromer, Joel R.
531 N. Charlotte St.
Pottstown, PA 19464
610-326-9797

Gottlieb, Richard
3347 Forbes Ave.
Pittsburgh, PA 15213
412-682-7017

Hendler, Barry H.
7901 Bustleton Ave., # 304
Philadelphia, PA 19152
215-333-0777

Holmes, John L.
98 Market St.
Mifflinburg, PA 17844
717-966-3333

Moser, Kem C.
415 McFarlan Rd.
Kennett Square, PA 19348
610-444-6300

Petrone, Joseph F.
3501 Terrace St.
Pittsburgh, PA 15261
412-648-8393

Phillips, John Q.
204 N. Main St.
Zelienople, PA 16063
724-452-9732

Rafferty, Thomas K.
209 Main St.
Latrobe, PA 15650
412-539-7781

Ramer, Elliot
419 Lawrence Rd.
Broomall, PA 19008
610-356-2400

Robbins, James L.
200 E. State St., # 103
Media, PA 19063
610-565-7200

Rogers, Robert R.
St. Barnabas Med. Ctr.
5830 Meridan Rd.
Gibsonia, PA 15044
724-444-4727

Smith, Stephen D.
Rt. 252 & Waynesborough
Rds.
Paoli, PA 19301
610-647-2755

Solga, Francis G.A.
103 E. Main St.
Schuylkill Haven, PA 17972
717-385-1344

Spiegel, Edward P.
3563 Aberdeen Rd.
Erie, PA 16506
814-833-1516

Zucker, Marc D.
826 Porter St.
Philadelphia, PA 19148
215-389-0380

RHODE ISLAND

Matrullo, Paul J.
1280 Park Ave.
Cranston, RI 02910
401-943-0644

Rosenberg, Cynthia L.
120 Dudley St., # 304
Providence, RI 02905
401-421-5600

Ross, Stuart
67 Jefferson Blvd.
Warwick, RI 02888
401-781-2742

SOUTH CAROLINA

Barbieri, Frank R.
3901 C Main St.
Hilton Head Island, SC
29926
803-689-2483

Began, Thomas J.
1507 Ebenezer Rd.
Rock Hill, SC 29732
803-327-1144

Burriss, J. Thomas
1000 Pinetop Rd.
Belton, SC 29627
864-338-6589

Crout, Danny K.
233 E. Blackstock Rd., # D
Spartanburg, SC 29301
864-576-3678

Dick, Douglas S.
1065 Johnnie Dodds Blvd.
Mount Pleasant, SC 29464
803-856-9323

Hanley, William J.
1203 Main St.
Hilton Head Island, SC
29926
803-681-6200

Kasparek, Gene A.
1507 Ebenezer Rd.
Rock Hill, SC 29732
803-328-2100

Kucaba, Walter J.
151 Dillon Dr.
Spartanburg, SC 29307
803-585-0468

Melchers III, J. Ted
1309 Warrick Lane
Mount Pleasant, SC 29464
803-881-0668

Merritt, Woodrow W.
514 Reed Rd.
Anderson, SC 29621
803-225-3141

Richardson, David W.
171 Ashley Ave.
Charleston, SC 29425
803-792-4451

Tysl, Ronald E.
121 River St.
Belton, SC 29627
864-338-8521

White, John R.
1352 A Cleveland St.
Greenville, SC 27607
864-271-4006

SOUTH DAKOTA

Lytle, Joseph M.
710 Mt. Rushmore Rd.
Rapid City, SD 57701
605-342-0977

TENNESSEE

Abrahamsen, Thomas C.
3100 Walnut Grove Rd.
Memphis, TN 38111
901-454-0660

Campbell, Jerry C.
800 Madison
Memphis, TN 38163
901-448-6930

Carney, Gilbert D.
6250 Poplar Ave.
Memphis, TN 38119
901-821-9922

Debow, Dwight A.
1203 N. Wilcox Dr.
Kingsport, TN 37664
423-247-5137

Pryse, John C.
180 Edgewood Ave.
Clinton, TN 37716
423-457-2299

Salmons, William K.
4329 Ball Camp Dr.
Knoxville, TN 37921
423-521-7707

TEXAS

Adams, Samuel H.
3735 Drexel, # C
Houston, TX 77027
713-623-2260

Blevins, Bryan O.
10 Med. Ctr., # H
Lufkin, TX 75904
409-634-1111

Bruenjes, Glen L.
909 Dairy Ashford, # 104
Houston, TX 77079
281-493-4173

Buehler, Stephen A.
3515 Ella Blvd.
Houston, TX 77018
713-682-4406

Collins, Scot F.
600 W. Hwy. 6
Waco, TX 76712
254-776-1575

Cuellar, Martin C.
13231 Champion Forest
Dr., # 304
Houston, TX 77069
713-444-2755

Denbar, Martin A.
3301 Northland Dr., # 400
Austin, TX 78731
512-454-8696

Fontana Jr., Vincent
207 W. Sunset
San Antonio, TX 78209
210-826-9523

Frantz, Don E.
400 Med. Ctr. Blvd., # 209
Webster, TX 77598
281-338-6631

Hancock, Larry B.
1125 University Dr.
Nacogdoches, TX 75961
409-564-2030

Hildinger, Michael D.
4402 Broadway Blvd., # 12
Garland, TX 75043
214-240-1781

Hinderstein, Barry
9099 Katy Fwy., # 180
Houston, TX 77024
713-932-0441

Holt, Charles R.
1100 Airport Freeway, # 206
Bedford, TX 76022
817-283-0025

Lucas, Edgar A.
Sleep Consultants, Inc.
1521 Cooper St.
Fort Worth, TX 76104
817-332-7433

May, James W.
2201 W. Holcombe, # 210
Houston, TX 77030
713-665-6886

Pritchard, Larry J.
7104 Sanger
Waco, TX 76712
817-751-1171

Roberts, D. Heath
8140 Walnut Hill Ln., # 100
Dallas, TX 75231
214-750-7776

Shirley, Joe E.
907 Bay Area Blvd.
Houston, TX 77058
713-488-5206

Smith, Robert A.
4800 N.E. Stallings
Nacogdoches, TX 75961
409-564-2417

Spence, Robert M.
5501 Independence Pkwy.
Plano, TX 75023
972-596-0200

Thomson, William K.
1010 Mopac Cir.
Austin, TX 78746
512-327-7930

Thornton, W. Keith
6131 Luther Lane, # 208
Dallas, TX 75225
214-691-5621

Washburn, Roy S.
3110 Webb St., # 300
Dallas, TX 75205
214-528-7870

VERMONT

Blanck, David R.
66 Colchester Ave.
Burlington, VT 05401
802-862-8348

McLaughlin, Donald
135 N. Main St.
Rutland, VT 05701
802-773-7000

Reiman, Edward K.
98 Merchants Row
Rutland, VT 05701
802-775-0300

VIRGINIA

Alexander, John M.
7650 Parham Rd., # 110
Richmond, VA 23233
804-270-5028

Bowler, Michael W.
4310 Geo. Washington
Hwy.
Yorktown, VA 23692
804-898-1919

Cherin, Jack I.
5101 Princess Anne Rd.
Virginia Beach, VA 23462
757-497-8611

Gregg, John M.
2727 S. Main St.
Blacksburg, VA 24060
540-951-8777

Hoard, Brian C.
Box 464 Dept. of Dentistry
Univ. of Virginia Med. Ctr.
Charlottesville, VA 22908
804-924-5005

McMunn, Michael O.
8804 Patterson Ave.
Richmond, VA 23229
804-740-7212

Nottingham, James H.
142 W. York St., # 705
Norfolk, VA 23507
804-623-9545

Rosenthal, Ron L.
408 East Market St.
Charlottesville, VA 22902
804-974-4646

Strauss, Arthur M.
311 Park Ave.
Falls Church, VA 22046
703-237-2350

Terwilliger, Gayle
501 Cedar Rd.
Chesapeake, VA 23320
757-548-0000

Waddell, Stacey L.
8804 Patterson Ave., # 100
Richmond, VA 23229
804-740-7212

WASHINGTON

Bales-Berg, Diantha J.
1216 N.E. 65th St.
Seattle, WA 98115
206-522-3300

Barrett, Patrick E.
19365 7th Ave. N.E., # 114
Poulsbo, WA 98370
360-779-7711

Carstensen, Steve
13401 Bel Red Rd., # A-6
Bellevue, WA 98005
425-746-0021

Choy, Eugene
1410 Meridian, S., # B
Puyallup, WA 98371
253-841-4341

Grim, Donald L.
3525 Ensign Rd., N.E., M-1
Olympia, WA 98506
206-456-6520

Halpin, E. Cary
13344 First Ave., N.E.
Seattle, WA 98125
206-364-8006

Horchover, Robert L.
1860 58th St., N.E.
Tacoma, WA 98422
253-927-7147

Hovorka, Daniel J.
1201 N. Garden St.
Bellingham, WA 98225
360-671-5671

Johnson, Robert E.
1149 Med. Dental Bldg.
Seattle, WA 98101
206-682-3888

Knutson, Larry B.
W. 101 Cascade Way, # 101
Spokane, WA 99208
509-468-0490

Larsen, John S.
1001 4th Ave., # 420
Seattle, WA 98154
206-554-7750

Lindblad, Randy E.
68 S.W. 13th St.
Chehalis, WA 98532
360-748-1833

Lloyd, Aaron D.
1135 N.W. Gilman Blvd.
Issaquah, WA 98027
425-392-6455

Marinkovich, Steven P.
5225 Tacoma Mall Blvd.
Tacoma, WA 98409
253-474-3223

Moore, Richard W.
2103 N.E. 272nd Ave.
Camas, WA 98607
360-834-9218

Paulin Jr., William B.
P.O. Box 3770
Silverdale, WA 98383
360-698-9335

Rohn, Delbert E.
S.E. 1205 Professional Mall
Pullman, WA 99163
509-332-2366

Seal, Thomas M.
9750 N.E. 120th Place
Kirkland, WA 98034
425-865-0937

WEST VIRGINIA

Szarko, James F.
2000 Dudley Ave.
Parkersburg, WV 26101
304-422-5177

WISCONSIN

Crowley, Robert J.
2450 S. Oneida St.
Green Bay, WI 54304
920-499-6244

Goetsch, Eugene R.
N63 W23669 Silver Spring
Dr.
Sussex, WI 53089
414-246-6806

Hack, Richard A.
2101 E. Calumet St.
Appleton, WI 54915
414-731-2773

Langyel, Eileen M.
3783 S. 108th St.
Greenfield, WI 53228
414-546-3424

Papandrea, James J.
10202 W. Hays Ave.
West Allis, WI 53227
414-321-2720

Slotnick, Jan H.
6789 N. Green Bay Ave.
Glendale, WI 53209
414-352-5650

Stevens, Christopher J.
425 W. Main St.
Sun Prairie, WI 53590
608-837-4880

Van Dyke, Robert J.
1551 Park Place
Green Bay, WI 54304
414-497-8500

Zernzach, Rudolph C.
325 E. Main St.
Winneconne, WI 54986
920-582-4344

CANADA

Anderson, Donald V.
3335 Dunbar St.
Vancouver, BC V6S 2B9
Canada
604-224-5611

Beach, Harold N.
312 Fairmont Ave.
Ottawa, ON K1Y 1Y8
Canada
613-728-5364

Clinton, Robert J.
4310 Stage Coach Rd.
Sydenham, ON K0H 2T0
Canada
613-376-6652

Cote, David
251 Blvd. St. Joseph
Hull, PQ J8Y 3X5
Canada
819-770-4944

Courtright, Patricia N.
#232, 4935 40th Ave. N.W.
Calgary, AB T3A 2N1
Canada
403-286-2399

Earl, Nancy A.
407-4935 40th Ave. N.W.
Calgary, AB T3A 2N1
Canada
403-247-2262

Goldberg, Y.K. Kenneth
7089 Younge St., # 203
Thornhill, ON L3T 2A7
Canada
905-731-1871

Halstrom, Wayne L.
503-805 W. Broadway
Vancouver, BC V5Z 1K1
Canada
604-875-0330

Hoffer, Marshall D.
2nd Floor, 191 River Ave.
Winnipeg, MB R3L 0B1
Canada
204-453-1788

Lawlor, Ken
18 Crown Steel Dr.
Markham, ON L6C 1G3
Canada
905-475-7600

Liem, Edmund K.T.
#3-5640 Vedder Rd.
Chilliwack, BC V2R 3M7
Canada
604-8584441

Lowe, Alan A.
Univ. of British Columbia
Faculty of Dentistry
2199 Wesbrook Mall
Vancouver, BC V6T 1Z3
Canada
604-822-3414

Luckhurst, Adrian C.
#14-1153 Esquimalt Rd.
Victoria, BC V9A 3N7
Canada
604-386-3044

Major, Paul W.
Rm. 5069C,
Dent/Pharmacy
Univ. of Alberta
Edmonton, AB T6G 2N8
Canada
403-492-7696

Mark, Jeffrey
Phase IV Dental Group
2 King St. W.
Hamilton, ON L8P 1A1
Canada
905-521-2181

Medock, M. Terry
290-11012 Macleod Trail
Calgary AB T2J 6A5
Canada
403-278-3444

Milroy, John D.
22 Richmond St., # 207
Richmond Hill, ON
L4C 3Y1
Canada
905-884-3713

Morisson, Florence M.
Univ. of Montreal
C.P. 6128 Centre Ville
Montreal QB J8C 3J7
Canada
514-343-6111

Pancer, Jeffrey P.
1621 Bloor St. W.
Toronto ON M6P 1A6
Canada
416-533-5440

Price, Barbara L.
420 Highway #7E,
Unit # 10
Richmond Hill, ON
L4B 3K2
Canada
905-882-0026

Priemer, Leslie P.
40 Sheppard Ave. W., # 100
North York, ON M2K 2W4
Canada
416-224-9998

Redigonda, Marco
2301 Major Mackenzie Dr.
Maple, ON L6A 1R8
Canada
905-832-5570

Rondeau, Brock H.
1275 Highbury Ave.
London, ON N5Y 1A8
Canada
519-455-4110

Roycroft, Brian E.
#101-10601 Southport Rdse.
Calgary, AB T2W 3M6
Canada
403-278-6664

Schachter, Maurice
#211-2535 Major Mackenzie
Dr.
Maple, ON L6A 1C6
Canada
905-832-3700

Stern, David J.
2 Conley St., # 2
Thornhill, ON L4J 7Z7
Canada
905-660-6658

Tan, Han-Kuang
4036 A Dentistry/
Pharmacy
Univ. of Alberta
Edmonton AB T6G 2N8
Canada
403-492-4471

Tyler, David W.
Univ. of Saskatchewan
107 Wiggins Rd.
Saskatoon, SK S7N 5E5
Canada
306-966-5135

Viviano, John S.
4099 Erin Mills Pkwy.
Mississauga, ON L5L 3P9
Canada
905-820-3200

Wechsler, Morris H.
5800 Cavendish Blvd.
Montreal, PQ H4W 2T5
Canada
514-486-1297

Woo, Stephen
4218 Lawrence Ave. East
Toronto, ON M1E 4X9
Canada
416-281-0882

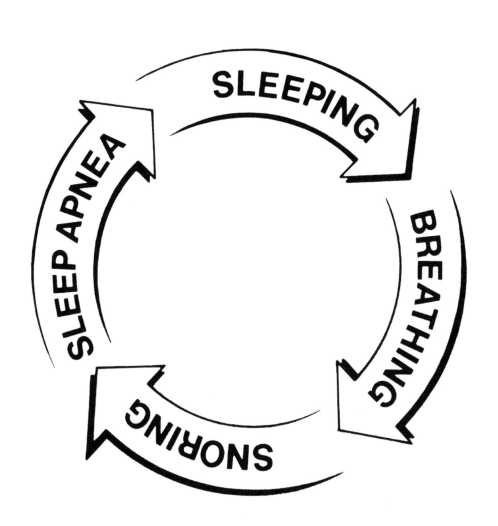

Here's the Easy Way to Order
Additional Copies of

Snoring Can Kill!!

The Ideal Gift for a Friend or Family Member

Phone orders: 800.450.3566 or 310.454.4333

Fax orders: 310.459.1575

E-mail orders: carenpublishing@worldnet.att.net

Internet orders: snoringcankill.com

Please send _____ (qty.) copies of *Snoring Can Kill!!* at $15.95 ppd each to:

Name: _____

Address: _____

City: _____ State: _____ Zip: _____ – _____

Tel: _____ E-mail: _____

Payment: ❏ Visa   ❏ MasterCard   ❏ Discover

Card Number: _____ Exp. date: _____ / _____

Name on card: _____

❏ Check by fax:

Make out check for correct amount, payable to Caren Publishing Group.

Fax your check to 310.459.1575. No need to mail check.

Sales tax to California addresses: 8.25%

Caren Publishing Group
1515 Palisades Drive, Suite M
Pacific Palisades, CA 90272

QUANTITY AND GROUP DISCOUNTS AVAILABLE